Recent Results in Cancer Research

Fortschritte der Krebsforschung
Progrès dans les recherches sur le cancer

49

Complications of Cancer Chemotherapy

Edited by

G. Mathé and R. K. Oldham

With 34 Figures

Springer-Verlag Berlin · Heidelberg · New York 1974

Proceedings of the Plenary Session of the European Organization for Research on Treatment of Cancer (E.O.R.T.C.) Paris, June 1973

GEORGES MATHÉ, Professor Institut de Cancérologie et d'Immunogénétique, Hôpital Paul-Brousse, F-94 Villejuif

ROBERT K. OLDHAM, M. D., Cellular and Tumor Immunology Section Department of Health, Education and Welfare, N.I.H. Bethesda, MD 20014/USA

Sponsored by the Swiss League against Cancer

Library of Congress Cataloging in Publication Data
Main entry under title:
Complications of cancer chemotherapy.
(Recent results in cancer research, 49)
"Proceedings of the Plenary Session of the European Organization for Research on Treatment of Cancer (E. O. R. T. C.), Paris, June 1973."
"Sponsored by the Swiss League against Cancer."
Bibliography: p.
1. Cancer-chemotherapy — Complications and sequelae — Congresses. I. Mathé, Georges, 1922— ed. II. Oldham, Robert K., ed. III. European Organization for Research into Treatment of Cancer. IV. Schweizerische Nationalliga für Krebsbekämpfung und Krebsforschung. V. Series. [DNLM: 1. Neoplasms — Complications. 2. Neoplasms — Drug therapy. W1RE106P v. 49/QZ267 M426ca]
RC261.R35 no. 49 [RC271.C5] 616.9'94'008s [616.9'94'061] 74-10820

ISBN-13:978-3-642-80850-0 e-ISBN-13:978-3-642-80848-7
DOI: 10.1007/978-3-642-80848-7

Contents

Introduction

G. MATHÉ and R. K. OLDHAM *

Institut de Cancerologie et d'Immunogénétique, Hôpital Paul Brousse, Villejuif

Since the last war, cancer chemotherapy has been the object of very intensive and expensive research. Nevertheless, its development has been very slow, and its ultimate potential is today somewhat in doubt.

In doubt because it does not cure any cancer patients except a) females carrying placental choriocarcinoma, a semi-allogenic tumor, in which case, cure may be influenced by immune rejection, and b) children suffering from Burkitt's tumor, where the probable reason for the cure is that all the neoplastic cells are in the cycle, which is a unique condition among all the human tumor varieties. Whether the long term survivors in acute leukemia, lymphomas, certain sarcomas and certain testicular tumors are "cures" will require longer follow-up.

The idea that chemotherapy does not cure most cancer patients because all their neoplastic cells are not in cycle has led to the use of drug combinations. Whatever they are, "cocktail combinations" which are made up of drugs given according to any timing, or scientific combinations, based on pharmacodynamics, pharmacokinetics or cell kinetics data, are more toxic than single drugs, and are all the more toxic as the number of drugs in the combination is increased.

Presented in this volume are papers dealing with the problem of toxicity resulting from chemotherapy of cancer. This toxicity ranges from the commoner examples of hematopoietic and organ toxicity to the less well understood immunological toxicity of these agents. Well illustrated in several papers is the continued problem of infectious complications during therapy which represents a combination of hematopoietic and immunological toxicities. Among short term side effects, hematological and immunological insufficiencies, mainly complicated by infections, are the most frequent and severe. Intermittent administration is a solution which allows hemopoietic and immune restoration during the intervals between cycles; aseptic environment reduces the toxic cost due to infections; white cell transfusions are the only means able to save very severely infected patients. Hemato-oncologic intensive care (i. c.) units are now as necessary as cardiologic or respiratory i. c. units.

Long term side effects are now better known as chemotherapy is over 15 years old. Cancerogenesis and especially leukemogenesis due to cancer chemotherapy agents is now proven, especially when combined with radiotherapy. It is probable that

* Present address: Cellular and Tumor Immunology Section, Laboratory of Cell Biology, National Cancer Institute, Bethesda, MD.

some Hodgkin's disease patients presenting a very localized neoplasia have been dangerously overtreated. Another long term effect is the induction of sterility in young people receiving chemotherapy. If we know nothing today about induction of genetic abnormalities in the offspring of non-sterile patients treated with chemotherapy, we have to consider them seriously for the future.

In addition to posing the problem of toxicity, several authors direct their attention in both a theoretical and practical manner to the pressing problem of modifying this toxicity before it becomes manifest in complications. We are perhaps on the verge of having the capability to "predict" these toxicities of drugs and drug interactions in a manner accurate enough to be applied clinically.

A problem alluded to in these presentations and one that is perhaps the most important for the future is the immunological toxicities of these drugs and drug combinations. As the therapy of cancer is on the verge of the widespread use of specific and non-specific immunological stimulation (i. e. "immunotherapy") in the treatment of residual disease after primary therapy (surgery, radiation and chemotherapy) and sometimes concomitantly with secondary therapy (i. e. especially chemotherapy), it is crucial that we understand the "toxic cost" of these agents on the immunological system we are trying to stimulate. Particularly important may be the temporal characteristics of this toxicity relative to the particular cell types in the immune systems responding to immunological stimulation. Some preliminary studies have indicated the timing of chemotherapy and immunotherapy must be correlated correctly for both to be optimally effective and it is in this area that future studies must be critically evaluated.

The final area of toxic cost discussed in this volume is the problem of carcinogenesis by these drugs. It is doubtless true these agents to induce malignancy in some of the patients. In fast growing cancers where the patient's chance of survival is very low (i. e. carcinoma of the lung), this is not a very crucial problem. On the other hand, in diseases such as Hodgkin's and non-Hodgkin's lymphomas, as well as carcinoma of the breast where the drugs are effective and/or the natural history of the disease is long, we must consider the "toxic cost" of the therapy as well as the therapeutic gain. It must be realized the follow-up of the patients "cured" of these cancers is short and we may be seeing only the tip of the iceberg of the cancer inducing properties of these drugs. Hence, continued surveillance of these patients is very basic to future clinical trials.

Thus, when prescribing a chemotherapy formula or formulating a protocol for a clinical trial, the ethical aspects as well as the long and short term scientific aspects must be considered.

Application of Large Animal Toxicology to the Qualitative and Quantitative Predication of Drug Toxicity in Man

S. K. CARTER

National Cancer Institute, N. I. H., Bethesda, MD

In the preclinical stage of drug development, the most crucial correlation of data obtained in animals with the expected effects in man is in the area of toxicology. It is the preclinical toxicologic evaluation of a new drug that enables the clinician to initiate clinical trial with a reasonable assurance of a safety margin for his patients.

Studies of large animal toxicology provide both a qualitative and quantitative prediction of the human experience. The qualitative aspects highlight the organ systems most likely to undergo damage and determine whether the toxic effects will be predictable, treatable and reversible. The quantitative information entails the choice of an initial dose for clinical trial and a prediction of the steepness of the dose response curve.

Considerable expertise in preclinical toxicology is available in the Drug Development Program of the Division of Cancer Treatment (DCT), in the National Cancer Institute, which for many years has evaluated all new drugs in the rhesus monkey and beagle hound before initiation of clinical trials. This review will consider some of this data within the DCT Cancer Therapy Evaluation Program (CTEP) from the standpoint of its potential for providing a qualitative and quantitative prediction of antitumor drug toxicology in man.

The Qualitative Approach

One of the most controversial areas in the development of new drugs for use in man involves the efficacy of animal toxicology as a predictive system for qualitative toxicity. The general approach of evaluating a new compound for safety in several animal species is performed in an attempt to generate information that may alert the clinical pharmacologist to potential hazards. The process requires extrapolation of toxicity data from one species to another, and implicit is the assumption that particular animal species have significant predictive value for toxicity in man and that important toxicity will not go unpredicted.

In order to meet the requirements of the United States Food and Drug Administration, all of the drugs in the DCT program are studied in the rhesus monkey and the beagle hound.

Our laboratory of toxicology uses a standard protocol including the following studies:

1. Single dose (dogs).
2. Five consecutive daily treatments (dogs—monkeys).
3. Five consecutive daily treatments, nine day rest; repeated for three treatment periods.
4. Schedule dependency studies in dogs on one of 3 schedules with the choice being based on schedule dependency results in leukemia L1210. These schedules are:

A. 48 hour infusion weekly for 6 weeks,
B. Treatment every 6 hours for 48 hours for 6 weeks,
C. Weekly treatment for 6 weeks.

The single dose schedule serves as a pilot study to permit the selection of an initial dose level for subsequent studies in dogs and monkeys, and to acquaint the investigator with the toxicologic potential of the drug under test.

The five daily dose treatment allows one to determine the toxicologic parameters to repeated administration of graded doses of the compound and to compare these with single treatment results.

The five daily treatments, followed by a 9-day rest, repeated for three treatments allow an estimation of the rate of recovery from drug toxicity and, hopefully, helps to determine the accumulative effects of the drug.

48 hour infusions or treatment every six hours are used for drugs that have schedule dependency in experimental tumor systems. These preclinical treatment schedules are intended to duplicate those to be used in Phase I clinical trials.

Weekly drug treatment is studied when it is felt that this schedule is likely to be used clinically.

Routinely, both male and female animals are included in each study group. Half of the animals are sacrificed 24 hours after the last treatment; the other animals are allowed at least 45 days following the last treatment to recover from drug effects or to demonstrate signs of delayed toxicity.

These studies provide the following information:

1. The highest nontoxic dose of a new agent in dogs and monkeys.
2. An indication of major organ toxicity in both species.
3. Evaluatión of predictability of toxicity.
4. Determination of reversibility of major toxicity.
5. Comparison of the consistency of quantitative and qualitative toxicity within and between species.
6. Determination of the influence of dosage schedule on drug toxicity.
7. Awareness of the possibility of delayed drug hazards.
8. Description of etiologic aspects of drug-induced toxicity as indicated by hematologic, chemical and histopathologic findings.

Recently, Dr. Phillip Schein and I reviewed the available data on 25 compounds of diverse and functional classification, in an attempt to see how well the combined dog and monkey screen predicted qualitative toxicities in man. These drugs included commonly used and well known compounds such as cytosine arabinoside, 5-fluorouracil, daunorubicin, mitomycin c, mithramycin, DTIC and BCNU, as well as lesser known compounds like dibromomannitol, streptozotocin, porfiromycin, hexamethylmelamine, azotomycin and 1-acetyl-2-picolinoyl hydrazine.

Fig. 1 outlines the percentage of the 25 drugs producing individual parameters of toxicities and our method of data analysis. As can be seen, a greater percentage of the drugs produced toxicity in animals than in man.

Percentage of drugs producing individual parameter toxicities

	Dog	Monkey	Man
Anemia	80	83	48
Leukopenia	72	74	80
Thrombocytopenia	72	30	76
Vomiting	96	30	84
Diarrhea	84	30	40
Alkaline Phosphatase ↑	76	24	32
SGOT ↑	60	56	44
Azotemia	64	65	36
Convulsion	20	0	4
Ataxia	44	17	12

Method of data analysis

	Animal	Man
TP — True positive	+	+
FP — False positive (overprediction)	+	−
TN — True negative	−	−
FN — False negative (underprediction)	−	+

Fig. 1. Prediction of qualitative toxicity from laboratory animals to man (Data of Schein, P. S., *et al.*, Laboratory of Toxicology, NCI)

The combination of dog and monkey as a toxicologic screen predicted myelosuppression by each of the 22 compounds that produced this toxicity in man. The total lack of false negatives, or underprediction, was the result of an overlap in information contributed by using the 2 species. The success is not so complete when individual parameters of myelosuppression are considered.

The combined animal screen predicted all drugs that produced anemia, but at the expense of 44% overprediction. The monkey and the dog performed equally well in predicting leukopenia with a 68% combined true positive. However, false negative results, or underprediction, which was not corrected by the combination, was found for both species. Table 1 lists those compounds in which one or both animal species failed to predict leukopenia. There are only 2 compounds for which both the dog and monkey failed to predict leukopenia, i. e., the progestational agent (NSC 17256E) and the antibiotic, Tubercidin. Both of these caused only a slight incidence of leukopenia in man, none of it severe. Because of the manner in which our program was written, any compound producing a toxic parameter in any patient caused that parameter to be listed as positive in man, even if the incidence was quite low.

Thrombocytopenia was correctly predicted for 13 of the 18 compounds causing this toxic effect in man. The compounds for which thrombocytopenia was not predicted are also shown in Table 1. The most serious failure was with mithramycin, which can cause severe thrombocytopenia. NSC 69945, a cyclophosphamide analogue, shares the platelet sparing effect of its parent compound but did cause platelet depression in a few patients.

The combined dog and monkey screen gave 92% true positives and no false negatives for gastrointestinal toxicity when compared with that of man.

Table 1. Compounds for which one or both animal species failed to predict leukopenia and thrombocytopenia

Compounds	Species that failed to predict for leukopenia in man	Species that failed to predict for thrombocytopenia in man
NSC 13875 Melamine, hexamethyl-	Monkey	Monkey
NSC 17256 E Pregn-4-ene-3,11,20-trione, 6 α-methyl-	Dog, monkey	—
NSC 19893 Uracil, 5-fluoro	—	Monkey
NSC 24559 Mithramycin (USAN)	Monkey	Dog, monkey
NSC 26980 Mitomycin C	—	Monkey
NSC 40774 9H-Purine, 6-(methylthio)-9-β-D ribofuranosyl-, dihydrate	Dog	Monkey (not measured in dog)
NSC 51095 Ammonium, trimethylpurin-6-yl-chloride	Monkey	Monkey
NSC 52947 Pactamycin	—	Monkey
NSC 53398 Restrictocin	—	Dog, monkey
NSC 56408 Tubercidin	Dog, monkey	—
NSC 62512 Acetophenone, 2-(dimethylamino)-3′,4′-dihydroxy-, hydrochloride	—	Dog, monkey
NSC 65346 Sangivamycin	Dog	—
NSC 69945 Phosphorodiamidic acid, N,N,-bis (2-chloroethyl)-, compd. with cyclohexylamine (1 : 1)	—	Dog, monkey

The prediction of gastrointestinal toxicity is outlined in Fig. 2. The most consistent clinical gastrointestinal toxicity induced by drugs was vomiting, which occurred with 18 of the 25 compounds. The combined screen gave 72% true positives, but missed 12% drug-related emesis. These results were primarily contributed by the dog, since there was significant underprediction in the monkey. For diarrhea, roughly the same situation was true.

	TP (%)	FP (%)	TN (%)	FN (%)
Vomiting				
Dogs	72	16	0	12
Monkeys	26	13	4	57
Dogs and monkeys	72	16	0	12
Diarrhea				
Dogs	36	40	20	4
Monkeys	13	26	35	26
Dogs and monkeys	36	44	16	4
Gastrointestinal toxicity				
Dogs	92	8	0	0
Monkeys	74	9	0	17
Dogs and monkeys	92	8	0	0

Fig. 2. Prediction of gastrointestinal toxicity

	TP (%)	FP (%)	TN (%)	FN (%)
BUN				
Dog	24	36	28	12
Monkey	18	46	18	18
Dog and monkey	24	52	12	12
Proteinuria				
Dog	9	73	18	0
Monkey	0	43	43	14
Dog and monkey	9	73	18	0
Renal toxicity				
Dog	32	56	4	8
Monkey	35	43	13	4
Dog and monkey	36	56	4	4

Fig. 3. Prediction of renal toxicity

The large animal screen gave 36% true positives for renal toxicity, as outlined in Fig. 3. Underprediction occurred in only 1 (4%) of 25 compounds, but there was a 56% overprediction. In general, no specific advantage could be attributed to use of either the dog or monkey. As can be seen, both blood urea nitrogen and proteinuria gave a high degree of overprediction. The high incidence of renal function abnormalities in animals had its counterpart in the renal histopathological changes which were documented in most animals.

Fig. 4 details the prediction of toxic effects in the liver. The combined screen predicted all instances of hepatotoxicity, but at the expense of a 48% overprediction. The comparison of dog and monkey failed to disclose a species selectivity. When individual parameters were analyzed the transaminase and alkaline phosphatase proved to be the most useful.

This study, which is reported more fully elsewhere (SCHEIN *et al.*, 1970) indicates that use of both dogs and monkeys is essential to adequate prediction. It is clear that toxicologic data collected in both species can forewarn the clinician of a useful proportion of the total spectrum of organ-specific and, with certain stated limitations, specific parameter toxicities that might be encountered. With the possible exception

	TP (%)	FP (%)	TN (%)	FN (%)
BSP				
Dog	28	50	5	17 (18)
Monkey	33	45	11	11 (9)
Dog and monkey	26	47	5	21 (19)
Alkaline phosphatase				
Dog	33	42	17	8 (24)
Monkey	15	10	40	35 (20)
Dog and monkey	32	50	16	12 (25)
SGOT				
Dog	28	39	22	11 (18)
Monkey	33	23	33	11 (18)
Dog and monkey	35	40	20	5 (20)
Prediction of liver toxicity				
Dog	52	44	4	0
Monkey	52	35	13	0
Dog and monkey	52	48	0	0

Fig. 4. Prediction of toxic effects in the liver

of central nervous system and dermal toxicity, all serious organ system toxicities are well predicted. This is accomplished in many cases at the expense of a high percentage of false positive predictions, but we feel that this degree of inefficiency in the system is justifiable. In order to demonstrate all possible qualitative toxicities, the animals must receive a dose spectrum including severely toxic and lethal doses. If the clinical use of the drugs in this analysis had been at more toxic dose levels than the estimated maximum tolerated dose, it is quite possible that the frequency of false positive predictions by the animal species would be significantly lower.

It is our feeling that the effective use of animal toxicologic data, coupled with careful monitoring, considered judgement and expectation by the physician, jointly serve to forewarn of the development of critical organ system toxicities during an initial Phase I trial.

The Quantitative Approach

The great difficulties inherent in the extrapolation to man of results obtained in animal studies have been recognized for many years. Since its inception, the Drug Development Program of the DCT- NCI, has grappled with these problems and gathered some of the most detailed information pertinent to their intelligent solution.

FREIREICH *et al.* (1966) first discussed the quantitative comparison of the toxic effects of 18 selected anti-cancer agents in mouse, rat, hamster, dog, monkey, and man. They found that the maximum tolerated dose (MTD) in man, on a mg/m^2 basis, was about the same as that in each animal species. On a mg/kg basis, the MTD in man was $^1/_3$ the MTD in rhesus monkeys and $^1/_2$ the MTD in dogs. The largest ratio of predicted dose/observed dose was 3 in one (thioTEPA) of the 18 agents. FREIREICH *et al.* concluded that it would be reasonable to estimate the human MTD (mg/m^2) from the preclinical toxicology in the mouse, rat, dog, monkey, and hamster and to start clinical cancer chemotherapy trials at about $^1/_3$ the predicted dose.

Currently, the DCT Laboratory of Toxicology reports the data on every schedule tested in large animals as four dose levels:

Highest Non-Toxic Dose (HNTD). The highest dose at which no hematologic, chemical, clinical or pathologic drug-induced alterations occur; doubling this dose produces the aforementioned alterations.

Toxic Dose Low (TDL). The lowest dose to produce drug-induced pathologic alterations in hematologic, chemical, clinical or morphologic parameters; doubling this dose *produces no lethality.*

Toxic Dose High (TDH). The lowest dose to produce drug-induced pathologic alterations in hematologic, chemical, clinical or morphologic parameters; doubling this dose *produces lethality.*

Lethal Dose (LD). The lowest dose to produce drug-induced death in any animals during the treatment or observation period.

In the choice of an initial dose for beginning Phase I studies in man, the DCT employs $^1/_3$ of the TDL observed in the most sensitive species.

Recently, it was thought worthwhile to evaluate the quantitative interspecies comparison among dogs, monkeys, and man for a series of 15 agents, which recently entered clinical trial, to determine the actual predictability of the new dose levels described above. While such a comparison clearly might not work for every drug, because of interspecies differences in pharmacologic disposition, it probably works often enough to make the analysis valuable.

All of the compounds chosen for study (Fig. 5) entered clinical trial within the last several years, most of them in the last 5 years. The data of the Laboratory of Toxicology studies on dogs and monkeys was searched in an attempt to identify the four dose levels. In all cases an effort was made to translate the dose schedules in the animals to the identical schedule used in man where the schedules were not identical. It was assumed that the toxicity of anticancer agents is cumulative, as shown in mice by GRISWOLD *et al.*, 1963 and also accepted in the work of FREIREICH *et al.*, 1966. For example a dose of $10\ mg/m^2/d \times 5$ in animals translated to $5\ mg/m^2/d \times 10$ or $1\ mg/m^2/d \times 50$.

The human MTD (mg/m^2) of each drug was compared, in mg/m^2 where possible, to 4 dose levels in the beagle and rhesus monkey described above. The quantitative comparison was made by determining the ratio of the human MTD to the various animal dose levels. Thus, if the ratio of the human MTD to a given animal dose is > 1, the human MTD dose is higher than the dose compared for in the animal, and man would be the more sensitive species, if the dose levels compared were considered comparable.

Urea, 1,3-bis (2-chloroethyl) nitroso- (BCNU; NSC 409962)
Urea, 1-(2-chloroethyl)-3-cyclohexyl-1-nitroso- (CCNU; NSC 79037)
Streptozotocin (NSC 85998)
Imidazole-4 (or 5)-carboxamide, 5 (or 4)-(3,3-dimethyl-1-triazeno)- (DTIC, ICT, DIC; NSC 45388)
Imidazole-4 (or 5)-carboxamide, 5 (or 4)-[3,3-bis-(2-chloroethyl)-1-triazeno]- TIC Mustard; NSC 82196)
Camptothecin (NSC 100880)
N,N-bis-(2-chloroethyl) aniline (Aniline mustard; NSC 18429)
Dibromodulcitol (NSC 104800)
2,2′-(9,10-anthrylenedimethylene)bis(2-thio-thiopseudourea), dihydrochloride, dihydrate (Pseudourea; NSC 56054)
β-2′-deoxythioguanoside (β-TGdR; NSC 71261)
Guanazole (NSC 1895)
5-hydroxy-picolinaldehyde, thiosemicarbazone (5HP; NSC 107392)
5-Azacytidine (NSC 102816)
Ara-6MP (NSC 406021)
Phenesterin (NSC 104469)

Fig. 5. Drugs used in the quantitative interspecies comparison

An example of the analysis for CCNU (NSC 79037) is shown in Table 2. The ratio of the human MTD to the TDL is 3.2 in dogs and 3.6 in monkeys, and man is apparently the less sensitive species at those dose levels. The initial dose chosen

Table 2. Quantitative interspecies comparison for single oral doses of CCNU

Dose level in animals	Dog		Monkey	
	mg/m^2	Human MTD [a] / animal dose	mg/m^2	Human MTD [a] / animal dose
HNTD	—	—	—	—
TDL	40	3.2	36	3.6
TDH	—	—	—	—
LD	200	0.65	—	—

[a] Human MTD = 130 mg/m^2; NCI-VA Phase I study used a modified Fibonacci sceardh scheme to escalate from 15 mg/m^2 to 130 mg/m^2 in 6 steps.

for clinical trial was $^1/_3$ the TDL (15 mg/m^2) and the NCI-VA Medical Oncology Service phase I study reached the human MTD in 6 steps using a modified Fibonacci search scheme for dose escalation.

Table 3 outlines the ratios obtained for 15 drugs in the beagle hound. In addition, LD/TDL ratio in the beagle is included as a possible representation of the steepness of the dose response curve. The last column of the table shows the number of steps it would have taken, in a modified Fibonacci search scheme approach, to reach the established MTD in man starting with $^1/_3$ the TDL in the beagle. This also could be considered a representation of the predictive value of the beagle for man.

When the ratio of the human MTD to the beagle TDL shown in Table 3 is considered in detail (Table 4), it is seen that three drugs (camptothecin, phenesterin, and

Table 3. Ratios of the human MTD to the various dose levels in the beagle for 15 anticancer agents

Drug	Ratio of human MTD to dose levels in beagle				Beagle LD / Beagle TDL	Estimated number of Fibonacci steps
	TDL	$^1/_3$ TDL	TDH	LD		
BCNU	10	30	—	2.5	4	11
CCNU	3.2	9.6	—	0.65	5	6
Streptozotocin	6.2	18.6	2.5	1.25	4	10
DTIC	1.6	4.8	0.8	0.4	4	4
TIC Mustard	3	9	1.5	0.75	4	4
Camptothecin						
Single dose	0.3	0.9	0.1	0.07	4$^1/_2$	0
Weekly	0.8	2.3	0.17	0.08	10	4
Daily × 5	1.6	4.8	0.37	0.2	8	11
Aniline mustard	5	15	0.34	0.17	30	8
Dibromodulcitol	3.4	10.2	0.9	0.45	8	6
Pseudourea	0.4	1.2	0.28	0.14	3	4
Phenesterin	0.8	2.4	0.04	0.02	33	2
β-TGdR	14	42	1.7	0.8	16	12
Guanazole	2	6	0.6	0.3	6	5
5HP	5.7	17.1	0.65	0.3	18	9
5-azacytidine	14	42	3.2	1.8	8	12
Ara-6MP	25	75	1.8	0.84	30	13

Table 4. Comparison of the ratio of the human MTD to the TDL in the beagle for 15 anticancer agents

Range of ratios [a]	Number of drugs	Percentage of drugs
0.1—1	3	20%
1—10	9	60%
> 10	3	20%

[a] Mean ratio = 6.5; median ratio = 3.4; range 0.3—25.

pseudourea) have a ratio < 1. This means that if the choice of the initial human dose had been made directly from the beagle TDL, this dose would have been in the clearly unacceptable range of toxicity. This 20% rate of failure of the beagle TDL for predicting an initial nontoxic dose when translating directly means that this approach would not be feasable. Nine drugs had a ratio between 1 and 10, and 3 drugs had a ratio > 10. The mean and median ratios for the 15 drugs are 6.5 and 3.4 respectively, with a range of 0.3—25.0.

When 1/3 the TDL in beagles is used to determine the ratio with the human MTD the situation improves considerably (Table 5). Only one drug, camptothecin, has a ratio of < 1 and when looked at in detail it is only < 1 by one of the three schedules

Table 5. Comparison of the ratio of the human MTD to 1/3 TDL in the beagle for 15 anticancer agents. Overall mean = 18.7; Overall median = 9.6

Range of ratios	Number of drugs	Percentage of drugs	Mean	Median
0.1—1	1	7%	0.9	0.9
1—10	7	46.5%	4.3	4.8
> 10	7	46.5%	36	18.6

Table 6. Quantitative interspecies comparison for camptothecin administered by three dose schedules

	Single dose (Human MTD = 120 mg/m²)		Weekly dose (Human MTD = 67 mg/m²)		Daily × 5 (Human MTD = 15 mg/m²)	
Dose levels in animals	Dog (mg/m²)	Ratio Human MTD	Dog (mg/m²)	Ratio Human MTD	Dog (mg/m²)	Ratio Human MTD
HNTD	—	—	—	—	—	—
TDL	375 [a]	0.32	80 [b]	0.84	9 [c]	1.6
TDH	1200	0.1	400	0.17	40	0.37
LD	1700	0.07	—	—	75	0.2

[a] 1/3 TDL = 125 mg/m² is toxic! (Actual Baltimore Cancer Research Center starting dose was 18 mg/m²).

[b] 1/3 TDL = 27 mg/m². Four steps in modified Fibonacci approach.

[c] 1/3 TDL = 3 mg/m². $\cong$ 11 steps in modified Fibonacci (NCI-VA started at 1.5 mg/m² and took 12 steps).

(Table 6) for which it is possible to make the analysis. Fortunately, the phase I trial at the NCI Baltimore Cancer Research Center started at a much lower dose (18 mg/m²) and trouble was avoided. The analysis shown in Table 5 gives us some confidence that 1/3 the TDL in the most sensitive animal species is a safe approach, although it cannot be considered absolutely safe.

When the ratio of human MTD to TDH of the beagle is examined (Table 7), all of the ratios are close to 1. The mean ratio is 1.03 and the median is 0.8, with a range of 0.04—3.2. Five drugs have a ratio > 1, while in 8 (62%) it is < 1, indicating that more than half the time the TDH would not be acceptable for direct translation to a safe initial dose. If we assume that the TDH in animals is the MTD, then more than half the time man is a more sensitive species.

Data in the rhesus monkey is available for only 6 drugs (Table 8), which probably limits any meaningful comparisons. The ratio of the human MTD to the 1/3 TDL

Table 7. Comparison of the ratio of the human MTD to the TDH in the beagle for 13 anticancer agents

Range of ratios [a]	Number of drugs	Percentage of drugs
> 1	5	38%
< 1	8	62%

[a] Mean = 1.03; median = 0.8; range = 0.04—3.2.

Table 8. Ratios of the human MTD to various dose levels in rhesus monkey for 6 anticancer agents

Drug	Ratio of human MTD to dose levels in monkey				Monkey LD / Monkey TDL
	TDL	1/3 TDL	TDH	LD	
CCNU	3.6	10.8	—	—	—
Streptozotocin	6.2	18.6	1.7	0.85	7.5
DTIC	0.38	1.14	0.19	0.09	4
Aniline mustard	—	—	—	—	8
Dibromodulcitol	0.66	1.9	0.15	0.07	9
Pseudourea	0.6	1.8	0.28	0.14	4
Mean	2.6	6.6	0.6	0.3	
Median	0.6	1.9	0.25	0.1	

is > 1 for all drugs tested, while the ratio of human MTD to monkey TDL is < 1 for 3 of 5 drugs, again emphazing the danger of using the TDL without fractionating it in the translation to man.

A comparison of the ratios for the beagle and monkey (Table 9) indicates that the monkey is apparently the more sensitive species overall, but the number of drugs tested in the monkey is quite small and this inference must be made with caution.

A more detailed analysis of quantitative comparisons, involving many more drugs and including rodent species, is in progress in the CTEP. The results will be the subject of a future report.

Table 9. Comparison of the ratios of human MTD to various dose levels in the beagle and rhesus monkey

Ratio	Mean		Median	
	Beagle	Monkey	Beagle	Monkey
$\frac{MTD}{TDL}$	6.5	2.6	3.4	0.6
$\frac{MTD}{1/3\ TDL}$	18.7	6.6	9.6	1.9
$\frac{MTD}{TDH}$	1.03	0.6	0.8	0.25
$\frac{MTD}{LD}$	0.67	0.3	0.3	0.1

References

FREIREICH, E. J., GEHAN, E. A., RALL, D. P., SCHMIDT, L. H., SKIPPER, H. E.: Quantitative comparison of toxicity of anticancer agents in mouse, rat, hamster, dog, monkey, and man. Cancer Chemother. Rep. **50**, 219 (1966).

GRISWOLD, D. P., LASTER, W. R., SNOW, M. Y., SCHABEL, F. M., SKIPPER, H. E.: Experimental evaluation of potential anticancer agents. XII Quantitative drug response of Sa 180, Ca 755, and leukemia L1210 system to a "standard list" of "active" and "inactive" agents. Cancer Res. (supp. part 2) **23**, 271 (1963).

SCHEIN, P. S., DAVIS, R. D., CARTER, S. K., NEWMAN, J., SCHEIN, D. R., RALL, D. P.: The evaluation of anticancer drugs in dogs and monkeys for the prediction of qualitative toxicities in man. Clin. Pharmacol. and Ther. **11**, 3 (1970).

Hematological Toxicity: Biological Basis*

L. M. VAN PUTTEN

Radiobiological Institute TNO, Rijswijk / The Netherlands

A shortage of leukocytes and platelets may be treated by transfusions, as will be discussed by others. A search for a more efficient treatment or prevention of haemopoietic failure after chemotherapy has not yielded a better treatment. Autologous bone marrow transplantation after single high dose cytostatic therapy was not a successful method to combat toxicity. The biological basis of bone marrow toxicity should be studied in more detail to find better means to combat it. A retrospective look for the reason why bone marrow transplantation failed, indicates that stem cell loss was not the cause of death after single dose chemotherapy. Animal studies confirm, that X-ray lethality but not the mortality after chemotherapy may be prevented by stem cell replacement.

Fig. 1 shows a comparison of a) survival time (plotted horizontally) and b) stem cell survival (plotted vertically) after exposure of mice to an LD_{50} of drugs or radiation. (Stem cell survival was estimated 16 hrs after subcutaneous injection of the drug and immediately or 24 hrs after exposure to X-rays.) It is evident that the mortality after exposure to the cytostatic drugs is not associated with a depression of the surviving stem cell number to a similar extent as after X-ray exposure. Other factors must be responsible for the lethal toxicity, or mortality occurs so early after chemotherapy that stem cell replacement will not lead to timely repopulation to permit survival of the mice. This seems to indicate that after a single dose of a cytostatic drug, stem cell survival is not critical and indeed in man stem cell replacement has generally not been effective after chemotherapy, whereas it has been found effective after irradiation or after late toxic aplasia (chloramphenicol; anti-epileptic drugs).

It is very difficult to evaluate the situation after multiple drug doses, both in man and in experimental animals. Data are lacking but the experimental data on fractionated X-ray exposure suggest that the efficacy of protection by bone marrow transplantation is progressively reduced as the X-ray dose is administered in an increasing number of daily fractions (VAN BEKKUM, 1963). Nevertheless there is no doubt that in animals and in mice death through haemopoietic failure may occur as a consequence of fractionated chemotherapy. Other factors than a simple shortage of haemopoietic stem cells may be involved: the simultaneous depletion of stem cells

* Parts of the work were carried out in programs of the EORTC Stem Cell Club and the EORTC Screening Pharmacology Group.

and maturating cells seems a logical consequence of repeated drug administration and in this respect different drugs may differ in their effects. Fig. 2 indicates the differences in the rate of recovery of CFU (spleen colony forming haemopoietic stem cells) in mice. Recovery is rapid after Vinblastine and Cyclophosphamide, somewhat slower after the Nitrosoureas (MCCNU) and very slow after Myleran. This is in contrast to the apparent effect on peripheral blood; it seems that after

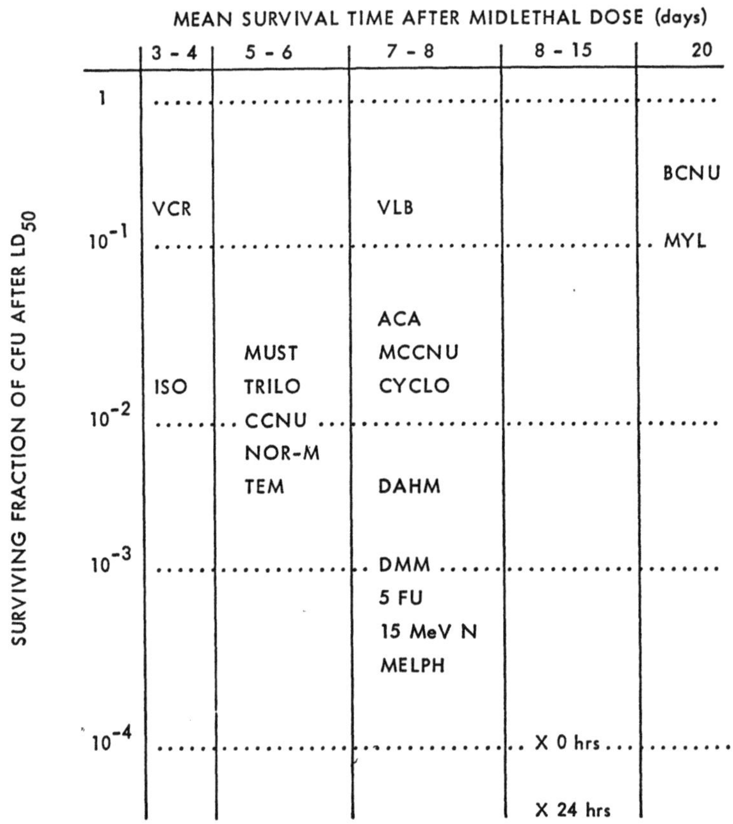

Fig. 1. Comparison of survival time and stem cell survival in mice exposed to drugs or irradiation at an LD50 dose. Drugs were administered subcutaneously and the survival of stem cells per femur was determined 61 hrs later in comparison with untreated controls. Stem cell survival was determined immediately and 24 hrs after exposure to X-rays. Details on mice and techniques for stem cell survival are given in VAN PUTTEN *et al.*, 1972

Myleran the prolonged depression of CFU numbers is not associated with a similarly delayed recovery of the peripheral blood. Perhaps the rate of proliferation of the exposed cells is decreased leading to a failure to recognize the CFU which form microcolonies in the spleen upon assay. The delayed depression is well-known for BCNU and CCNU, and the chronic depression and aplasia is a late sequel especially after Myleran. The mechanism of these delayed toxic effects are not clear and should be studied in more detail.

Of course the delay in recovery of haemopoiesis is important for the selection of optimal treatment schedules. Some information is available on other cytostatic drugs for which the spacing of drug doses is based on bone marrow depression. The Vinca alkaloids are usually given a weekly intervals and this is based on the greater haemopoietic toxicity of divided doses compared with a single dose. This is a consequence of the fact that the first dose of these drugs will kill a number of proliferating bone marrow cells followed by the recruitment of initially resting haemopoietic stem cells into rapid proliferation.

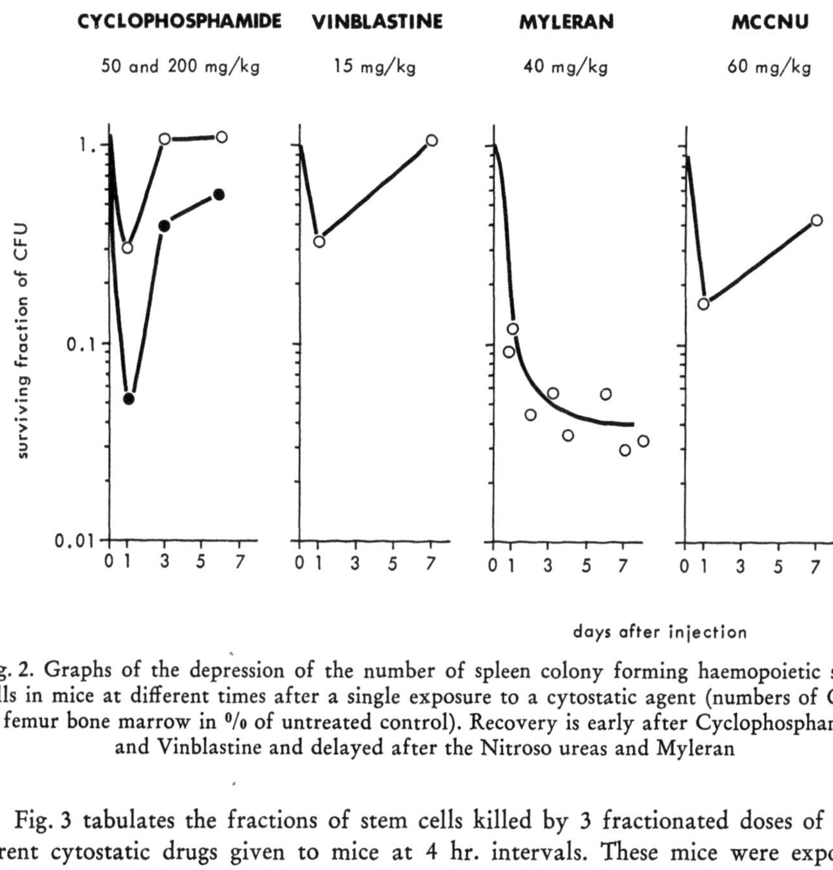

Fig. 2. Graphs of the depression of the number of spleen colony forming haemopoietic stem cells in mice at different times after a single exposure to a cytostatic agent (numbers of CFU in femur bone marrow in % of untreated control). Recovery is early after Cyclophosphamide and Vinblastine and delayed after the Nitroso ureas and Myleran

Fig. 3 tabulates the fractions of stem cells killed by 3 fractionated doses of different cytostatic drugs given to mice at 4 hr. intervals. These mice were exposed under two conditions: a) with stem cells resting and b) with stem cells in rapid proliferation after depletion by radiation. From other studies it is known that these drugs kill cells only when in cycle and thus we can calculate what fraction of the "resting" stem cells is seemingly in cycle.

A comparison with tritiated thymidine in vitro (^{3}HTdR, 20 min. exposure) shows that initially these stem cells are not in cycle and that they must have been recruited into cycle during the fractionated exposure. This recruitment into cycle sensitizes the cells to further exposure to cytostatic drugs and this may greatly contribute to the bone marrow toxicity of divided doses of cytostatic agents. It would be extremely useful if we could temporarily block this recruitment of stem cells. In this field some progress has been made. Byron has shown that neurotransmitters can induce resting stem cells to enter S-phase *in vitro* (Byron, 1972; Byron, 1973). Bruce *et al.* 1970 have shown that light anaesthesia with halothane can indeed partially protect mouse stem cells against the toxic effect of fractionated chemotherapy without simultaneous protection of leukaemic cells.

	Fraction of cells killed		
	Resting CFU (a)	Rapidly proliferating CFU (b)	Fraction of "resting" CFU seemingly in cycle (a/b)
Vinblastine	.81	.992	.82
Vincristine	.78	.993	.79
VM 26	.91	.995	.91
Hydroxyurea	.60	.992	.60
Procarbazine	.73	.98	.75
Emetine	.55	>.99	.56
Methotrexate	~0	~0	estimate impossible
6 Mercaptopurine	.78	.89	estimate impossible
Azathioprine	.62	.80	estimate impossible
Cytosine Arabinoside	.76	.992	.77
^{3}HTdR in vivo	.35	.992	.35
^{3}HTdR in vitro (20 min exposure)	.06	.57	.11

Fig. 3. Table indicating CFU killing by repeated exposure *in vivo* (3 doses at 4-hrs intervals) to cell cycle phase specific cytostatic drugs. The animals were exposed to the maximal tolerated doses of the agents. Resting CFU should not be affected as is indicated by the effect of tritiated thymidine in vitro (bottom line) whereas rapidly proliferating CFU are reduced by more than 99% after exposure to effective drugs. This permits an estimate of the fraction of CFU in cycle in the period of exposure. This is given in the fourth column (except for Methotrexate 6 Mercaptopurine and Azathioprine, which kill less than 90% of rapidly proliferating CFU). It is clear that the cytostatic drugs, especially the spindle poisons must recruit a large fraction of the CFU into cycle

At the last meeting of the EORTC Stem Cell Club Keizer reported that barbiturates can block the entry of resting stem cells into S-phase after X-ray exposure. On the basis of these data a project group of the Stem Cell Club is studying whether drugs that block neurotransmitters may be useful in the protection against bone marrow toxicity associated with chemotherapy. At this stage it is impossible to predict whether this approach will lead to an effective procedure in man, but it is clear that the recruitment of resting tumour cells into cycle which is necessary to achieve effective tumour cell killing, cannot be performed without simultaneously inducing resting haemopoietic stem cells to enter the cell cycle and thus making the haemopoietic system more sensitive to the toxic effects of chemotherapy.

References

BEKKUM, D. W. VAN: Foreign bone marrow transplantation following fractionated whole-body irradiation in mice. In: Radiation effects in physics, chemistry and biology, p. 362 (Ed.: M. EBERT and A. HOWARD), Amsterdam: North Holland Publishing Co. 1963.

BRUCE, D. L., LIN, H. S., BRUCE, W. R.: Reduction of colony-forming cell sensitivity to arabinyl cytosine by halothane anaesthesia. Cancer Res. **30**, 1803 (1970).

BYRON, J. W.: Evidence for a β-adrenergic receptor initiating DNA synthesis in haemopoietic stem cells. Exp. Cell Res. **71**, 228 (1972).

BYRON, J. W.: Drug receptors and the haemopoietic stem cell. Nature New Biol. **241**, 152 (1973).

PUTTEN, L. M. VAN, LELIEVELD, P., KRAM-IDSENGA, L. K. J.: Cell-cycle specificity and therapeutic effectiveness of cytostatic agents. Cancer Chemother. Reports Part 1, **56**, 6 (1972).

Abbreviations

VCR = Vincristine, VLB = Vinblastine, BCNU [1] = Bis-Chloro-aethyl Nitroso Urea, Myl [2] = Myleran (Busulfan), Iso [3] = Isophosphamide, MUST = Mechlorethamine, Trilo [3] = Trilophosphamide, CCNU [1] = Cyclohexyl-Chloroethyl-Nitroso-Urea, Nor-M = Bis-chloro-ethylamine, TEM [5] = Triethylene Melamine, ACA [6] = Aminochlorambucil, MCCNU [1] = Methyl-Cyclohexyl-Chloroethyl Nitroso Urea, Cyclo [3] = Cyclophosphamide, DAHM = Di-AnHydro-Mannitol [7], DMM = Di-Methyl-Myleran [7], 5FU [4] = 5 Fluoro-Uracil, 15 MeV N = 15 MeV neutron irradiation, Melph = Melphalan, X = 300 keV X-rays.

CFU = haemopoietic spleen colony forming stem cell, ^{3}HTdR = tritiated thymidine (9 Ci/mMol.), VM 26 = 4-demethyl-epipodophyllotoxin-thenylidene glucoside, supplied by Sandoz.

[1] Gift from the Drug Evaluation Branch, N.I.H.
[2] Gift from Wellcome Foundation.
[3] Gift from Asta Werke.
[4] Gift from Hoffmann-La Roche.
[5] Gift from Lederle.
[6] Gift from Mack for EORTC.
[7] Gift from Chester Beatty Research Institute.

Immunological Toxicity of Cancer Chemotherapy*

G. W. SANTOS

Department of Medicine, John Hopkins University, Baltimore, MD

The effective use of modern anti-cancer agents is always associated with some toxicity. Various forms of toxicity such as that directed toward the kidney, liver and bone marrow can often be easily measured and quantitated. The physician through experience is able to avoid irreversible toxicity by careful monitoring of several laboratory parameters. Toxicity to the immune system on the other hand is not easily measured although the consequences of profound immunosuppression in terms of increased susceptibility to viral, protozoal and fungal infections are well known.

In an admittedly oversimplified way, one can view the immune response as being initiated when antigen is processed by the macrophage system. This is followed by an interaction with the lymphoid system that leads to the proliferation and differentiation of lymphocytes to become sensitized cells capable of expressing cellular immunity or differentiation to plasma cells capable of secreting specific antibody. Sensitized lymphocytes and/or humoral antibodies together with complement act on the target antigen with the release of lymphokines, etc. The resulting tissue inflammation may further magnify the specific immunological events.

It is clear, therefore, that this very complex immune response may be affected at many different places. Although our knowledge of the effects of anti-cancer agents are limited in detail, certain principles have emerged. Several years ago we proposed an operational classification of anti-cancer agents (SANTOS, 1967).

Operational Classification of Drugs

Class I agents are most effective in suppressing the immune response when given just prior to the immune stimulus and relatively ineffective when given after. These agents act on early stages of the immune response that may have to do with antigen recognition, processing or informational transfer. Examples of such agents are ionizing radiation, melphalan, mitomycin C and cortisone.

Class II agents are most effective as immunosuppressants when given a day or two following the immunogenic stimulus and are ineffective if given before immunization. These agents for the most part are the cycle dependent drugs and affect the

* Supported by U.S. Public Health Service Grant No. CA-06973.

stages of proliferation and differentiation. Some of the agents in this class are mechlorethamine, chlorambucil, 6-mercaptopurine, azathioprine, methotrexate, actinomycin D, 5-fluorouracil, cytosine arabinoside, vinblastine and vincristine.

Class III agents are those agents that share properties with both Class I and II and are able to suppress the immune response when given either before or after the immunizing event. Cyclophosphamide and procarbazine are examples of this class. It should be noted that cyclophosphamide is most effective as an immunosuppressant when given after the immunization but, nevertheless, is quite effective when given just before immunization.

Differential Effects on IgM and IgG Antibody Formation

The primary antibody response is classically made up of an initial production of IgM antibody. When IgM levels reach their peak, IgG antibody appears and coincident with increasing levels of this class of antibody, IgM levels fall. A variety of Class I, II and III agents, under appropriate conditions, are able to preferentially suppress the IgG response. Elsewhere (SANTOS, 1972) we have argued that the "switch" mechanism of IgM to IgG antibody production is the most sensitive phase of the primary antibody response to the action of cytotoxic agents.

Drug-induced Immunological Tolerance

This important phenomenon originally described a number of years ago (SCHWARTZ and DAMESHAK, 1959) has been confirmed in a number of animal systems and in man (MAKINODAN *et al.*, 1970). Antigen given prior to the administration of Class II or III agents "selects" that system of immunocompetent cells that are capable of responding to the antigen, and set into motion the proliferative and differentiative stages of the immune response. If the agent is given at this time, it finds the cells involved in the immune response most sensitive to their cytotoxic action. Other clones of immunocompetent cells that have not been "turned on" by the antigen are relatively resistant. If the original "loading" antigen is given again with a second antigen after drug treatment has stopped, there is an immune response only to the new antigen, presumably because the clones of immunocompetent cells that could have responded to the original antigen have been eliminated or at least severely damaged.

The Adjuvant Effect of Immunosuppressive Drugs

Under certain conditions and in particular with the administration of Class II drugs just prior to immunization, an augmented immune response may be seen in both animals and in man.

The administration of the drug will be destructive to a variety of dividing cell populations such as hematopoietic cells and gut epethelial cells. If now the drug is stopped and an antigen is given, the normally resting (not in cycle) immunocompetent cells that have escaped the cytotoxic action of the cycle dependent drugs are able to respond to the antigen in a millieu of the products of cell destruction with an exaggerated response. Direct evidence for the hypothesis that products of cell destruction may behave as adjuvants has been reported (BRAUN, 1965).

Infections as a Result of Immunological Toxicity

The clinical infections with gram positive and negative bacteria associated with the administration of cytotoxic agents are in the main related to granulocytopenia rather than immunosuppression. Indeed, normal immune responses or even augmented responses may be seen immediately following short bursts of intensive chemotherapy.

It appears that immunosuppression is least when treatment with cytotoxic agents is given intensively in bursts at various intervals rather than in a more sustained and chronically maintained manner. Under the latter conditions immunosuppression may be marked and it is in just this setting that one sees the increased frequency of viral, fungal and protozoal infections. While these infections are most often related to a generalized immunosuppression it is quite possible that under certain conditions exposure to these various organisms at the "correct" time in relation to drug administration could result in specific tolerance to an infectious agent.

Toxic Effects on the Tumor Host Relationship

In the past several years, considerable evidence has accumulated that human tumors possess tumor specific antigens. Furthermore, often a given individual can be demonstrated to have cellular and humoral immunity to this or her own tumor *in vitro*. These observations have naturally excited clinicians who wish to use immunological means for therapy. Unfortunately, at present, there is a large gap in our knowledge as far as translating these *in vitro* observations to useful clinical principles. Work of perhaps a more fundamental nature in defined animal systems indicates that despite tumor immunogenicity there are a number of avenues of escape that a tumor may utilize. At present our knowledge in this area is rudimentary.

An oversimplification of what is known is perhaps useful for purposes of discussion. One can consider a given individual with cancer as having either good, weak, or absent cellular immunity to his or her tumor. The individual may or may not possess cytotoxic antibody and may or may not demonstrate blocking factors in his serum (humoral factors that block cell mediated immunity).

Theoretically, chemotherapy might change a given balance of these several factors that would lead to tumor enhancement or tumor destruction. If a particular treatment is generally immunosuppressive, one might expect that the degree and duration of the beneficial effects of anti-cancer treatment to be lessened and shortened. On the other hand, anti-tumor effects might be augmented if the immunosuppressive effect were to be greatest on humoral as opposed to cellular immunity.

A variety of agents are capable of "breaking" immunological tolerance and it is possible that such a mechanism could add to an anti-tumor effect. Conversely the situation might be reversed if tolerance was induced to tumor antigens.

It must also be remembered that under certain conditions anti-cancer treatment may produce adjuvant effects. This could lead to a better anti-tumor effect if, for instance, cellular immunity was increased preferentially. It is equally possible, however, that humoral responses often associated with blocking factors could be preferentially increased.

All of the above situations would seem possible. When we have data on *in vitro* monitoring by a variety of tests on patients throughout the history of their disease we will perhaps be able to make the meaningful correlations that will allow us to more rationally design both our approaches to chemotherapy and immunotherapy.

References

BRAUN, W. E.: Influence of nucleic acid degradation products on antibody synthesis. Molecular and cellular basis of antibody formation. p. 525. J. STERZL, Ed., New York: Academic Press 1965.

MAKINODAN, T., SANTOS, G. W., and QUINN, R. P.: Immunosuppressive drugs. Pharmacol Rev. **22**, 189 (1970).

SANTOS, G. W.: Immunosuppressive drugs I. Fed. Proc. **26**, 907 (1967).

SANTOS, G. W.: Chemical Immunosuppression. Transplantation p. 206. J. S. NAJARIAN and R. L. SIMMONS, Eds. Philadelphia: Lea and Febiger 1972.

Bacterial and Fungal Infections During Cancer Chemotherapy*

V. Rodriguez, G. P. Bodey **, and E. J. Freireich

Department of Developmental Therapeutics, The University of Texas
M. D. Anderson Hospital and Tumor Institute at Houston, Houston, TX

The cancer patient is susceptible to infection due to a complex interplay between his tumor and its therapy. Patients with hematological malignancies often have neutropenia, lymphopenia and impairment in antibody production and cellular immunity due to their neoplastic disease. Patients with solid tumors may have impairment of host defense mechanisms as their disease progresses. In addition tumor masses may become necrotic, or may obstruct drainage from body sites resulting in infection. Most antitumor agents also cause myelosuppression, immunosuppression and ulceration of the gastrointestinal tract which facilitates invasion by enteric organisms. The use of combination chemotherapy has increased our capabilities of treating patients with extensive malignancies but has also increased their susceptibility to infectious complications. As better modalities of cancer therapy become available, the diagnosis and management of infections will become increasingly important.

Infection is the major cause of death in cancer patients. This has been demonstrated repeatedly in patients with acute leukemia (Hersh *et al.*, 1965). We have recently investigated the causes of death in solid tumor patients and demonstrated that infection is also the major cause of death in such patients (Rodriguez *et al.*, 1973). The study was undertaken in 816 cancer patients who expired between Jan. 1968 and Dec. 1970 and had a complete post mortem examination. Infections caused death in 47% of the patients (Table 1). Other causes of death were organ failure, carcinomatosis, infarction and hemorrhage. Pneumonia accounted for 51% of the 380 fatal infections. It occurred mainly in patients with carcinomas of the lung, head and neck and melanomas. Septicemia accounted for 38% of infections and was most frequently found in patients with malignancies of the genitourinary and gastrointestinal tracts. Half of the patients with septicemia had other major infection. Peritonitis, pyelonephritis and meningitis accounted for most of the remaining infections. The infecting organisms were identified in 221 of the 380 infections (Table 2). The majoritiy were gram-negative bacteria. *E. coli, Pseudomonas aeruginosa* and *Klebsiella* sp. were the most frequent pathogens. *Bacteroides* spp. accounted for 8%

* Supported in part by Grant No. CA-10042 from the National Cancer Institute, National Institutes of Health, U.S. Public Health Service, Bethesda, MD.

** Dr. Bodey is a Scholar of the Leukemia Society of America, Inc.

of the organisms identified. Infections caused by gram-positive organisms, mixed flora or non-bacterial organisms occurred infrequently. There were 13 fungal infections in this study.

During the 2 weeks prior to death, 134 of the 816 patients received cancer chemotherapy and 61 of them died of infection (43%). Hence, the frequency of fatal

Table 1. Infections causing death in cancer patients

Type	Number patients	% of infections	% of total PTS
Pneumonia	192	51	24
Septicemia [a]	147	38	18
Peritonitis	25	6	3
Other [b]	16	5	2
Total	380	100	47

[a] Includes: Septicemia alone (72) and Septicemia plus other infections (75).
[b] Includes: Pyelonephritis (10), Meningitis (4), Tetanus (1), Viral Hepatitis (1).

Table 2. Organisms causing fatal infections

Type	Number		%	
Gram-negatives only		151		68
E. coli	50		23	
Pseudomonas aeruginosa	25		11	
Klebsiella	21		9	
Proteus sp.	19		8	
Enterobacter-serratia	17		8	
Bacteroides	17		8	
Other gram-negatives	2		1	
Gram-positive only		20		9
Staph. aureus	9		4	
Clostridia	5		2	
Other gram-positives	6		3	
Multiple organisms (mixed gram-positive and gram-negative)		34		15
Other [a]		16		7

[a] Fungi 13; M. Tuberculosis 2; Pneumocystis carinii 1.

infection was no greater among the group of patients receiving chemotherapy than among the group who were not receiving chemotherapy. The majority of fatal infections in the 816 patients were caused by tumor masses (67%) whereas only 14% were related to neutropenia, which was usually a side effect of chemotherapy. Since the majority of infections in these solid tumor patients resulted from the effects of tumor, better modalities of cancer therapy are needed for these patients before a major reduction in infectious complications can be accomplished.

We have reviewed the frequency of septicemia in cancer patients at our institution during a 3 year period (BODEY, 1971). There were 2.4 episodes per 100 hospital admissions among patients with solid tumors compared to 45 episodes among patients with leukemia. Gram-negative bacilli accounted for nearly 85% of these infections. The most common organisms were *E. coli, Klebsiella* spp. and *Ps. aeruginosa.* Patients hospitalized for treatment of leukemia acquired *Ps. aeruginosa* from the hospital environment. Those patients who become carriers of this organism are at much greater risk of developing Pseudomonas infection than those patients who do not become carriers.

We have monitored the microbiological flora of 34 leukemic patients during induction chemotherapy and studied its relationship to infections (RODRIGUEZ *et al.*, unpublished). Specimens of throat and stools were cultured from these patients on admission and weekly thereafter. Typing of *Ps. aeruginosa, E. coli* and *Klebsiella* sp. was done. The patients received systemic antibiotic therapy for fever due to presumed or proven infection with carbenicillin alone or in combination with cephalothin, kanamycin or gentamicin. Hospitalization periods ranged from 19—115 days with a median of 53 days. Less than a third of the aerobic bacteria cultured from throat and less than half of aerobic bacteria cultured from the stools on admission were no longer cultured during hospitalization. 69% of anaerobic bacteria cultured on admission from the throat and 48% cultured from stool also were no longer cultured (Table 3). During hospitalization newly acquired organisms were cultured from throat and stool specimens from all patients. Gram-negative aerobes, anaerobes and fungi were most prevalent.

Table 3. Monitoring of microbial flora in leukemia patients during chemotherapy

Organisms	Sites	Isolated initially	No longer cultured during hospitalization (%)	Newly acquired during hospitalization (%)
aerobes: gram (+)	throat	91	30	53
aerobes: gram (−)	throat	29	21	39
anaerobes	throat	16	69	8
fungi	throat	5	40	8
aerobes: gram (+)	stool	43	26	55
aerobes: gram (−)	stool	96	50	132
anaerobes	stool	33	48	59
fungi	stool	23	26	29
Total		336	38	383

Twenty of the 34 patients studied developed 27 episodes of infection. Nine of the infections were caused by organisms cultured from the patients on admission to the hospital. 12 infections were caused by organisms which were acquired by the patients during their hospitalization for antileukemic chemotherapy. Four infections were caused by organisms not cultured from the patient previously and in 2 infections the causative organism could not be identified. Twenty-two of the infections were caused by gram-negative bacilli. None were caused by anaerobes or fungi. Hence, over one-half of the infections were caused by organisms which were nosocomial in origin.

The types of infections occurring in cancer patients and their prognosis has changed substantially during the past 2 decades. For many years staphylococcal infections were a major problem in cancer patients. The introduction of the anti-staphylococcal semi-synthetic penicillins has virtually eliminated this problem. The development of gentamicin and carbenicillin has significantly improved the outcome of some gram-negative bacilli infections. For example, carbenicillin has increased the cure rate in Pseudomonas infections among cancer patients to greater than 80% whereas it had been only 24% with the polymyxins (BODEY *et al.*, 1971). Gentamicin has proven to be life-saving in the treatment of patients with infections caused by a strain of *Serratia marcesens* which is resistant to all other currently available antibiotics and has been responsible for micro-epidemics in our institution (BODEY *et al.*, 1970). However, in spite of advances in antimicrobial therapy the overall incidence of infections in cancer patients has not decreased substantially.

The increasing incidence of fungal infections in patients with cancer has been recognized during recent years. In a study of 454 patients with acute leukemia, 189 fungal infections were found at autopsy in 161 patients (BODEY, 1966). The yearly frequency of fungal infections increased from 10% to greater than 30% during a 10 year period. *Candida* sp. accounted for the majority of these infections. In our institution the incidence of serious fungal infections is less than 10% in patients with solid tumors, about 10% in patients with lymphomas and 25% in patients with acute leukemia. However, the overall incidence of fungal septicemia has increased from 2%—6% during the last 5 years. Various factors are responsible for the development of such infections. Among them are impaired immunological defenses, usage of broad spectrum antibiotics, corticosteroid therapy, indwelling catheters and intravenous hyperalimentation.

Unfortunately, the majority of serious fungal infections are seldom diagnosed antemortem due to the lack of specific signs and symptoms. Isolation of *Candida* spp. from clinical specimens is seldom helpful in establishing the diagnosis because the organism is so ubiquitous. The organism is cultured from blood specimens of only 25% of patients with disseminated candidiasis. Serological tests are being investigated but often are not helpful in the individual patient whose antibody titer fails to rise because of impaired immunological mechanisms. Aspergillosis and phycomycosis are rarely diagnosed antemortem because the organism is cultured infrequently from these patients. The cryptococcal antigen test has proven to be very useful in diagnosing cryptococcosis in cancer patients. Unfortunately, the treatment of systemic fungal infections in cancer patients is seldom successful unless the patient achieves a remission of his malignancy.

In summary, infections constitute the major complication during cancer chemotherapy and the most frequent cause of death in patients with neoplasias. Gram-negative bacilli are still the most frequent pathogens causing infections, but the prevalence of these pathogens has been altered with the effectiveness of new antibiotics. The incidence of fungal infections has also increased in cancer patients during recent years. The recognition and management of these infections constitutes an integral part of the present therapy of cancer patients. In fact, fatal infections in cancer patients are mainly produced by the underlying tumor rather than myelosuppressive effects of the antineoplastic therapy. Consequently, better modalities of supportive care but also more effective antineoplastic therapy are needed.

References

BODEY, G. P.: Fungal infections complicating acute leukemia. J. Chron. Dis. **19**, 667 (1966).

BODEY, G. P.: Infections and cancer: Natural history, diagnosis and treatment. In: Eds.: R. L. CLARK, R. W. CUMLEY, J. E. McCAY, and M. M. COPELAND. Oncology 1970, Being the Proceedings of the Tenth International Cancer Congress. Volume III: Diagnosis and Management of Cancer: General Considerations, p. 445. Chicago, Illinois: Year Book Medical Publishers, Inc. 1971.

BODEY, G. P., RODRIGUEZ, V., and SMITH, J. P.: *Serratia* species infections in cancer patients. Cancer (Philad.) **25**, 199 (1970).

BODEY, G. P., WHITECAR, J. P. JR., MIDDLEMAN, E., and RODRIGUEZ, V.: Carbenicillin therapy of pseudomonas infections. J. Amer. Med. Ass. **218**, 62 (1971).

HERSH, E. M., BODEY, G. P., NIES, B. A., and FREIREICH, E. J.: Causes of death in acute leukemia. A ten-year study of 414 patients from 1954—1963. J. Amer. Med. Ass. **193**, 105 (1965).

RODRIGUEZ, V., BODEY, G. P., and TURCK, M.: Changes in microbial flora of patients receiving antileukemic therapy. To be published.

RODRIGUEZ, V., INAGAKI, J., and BODEY, G. P.: Causes of death in patients with non-hematological malignancies (Abstract). American Society of Clinical Oncology, Ninth Annual Scientific Meeting, No. 54. Atlantic City, N. J., April 1973.

A Study of Viral Infections in Patients Treated with a Combination of 6 Mercaptopurine-Methotrexate: Preliminary Results

C. Jasmin [1], F. Bricout [2], J. M. Huraux [2], R. Weiner [3], R. K. Oldham [4] and G. Mathé [1]

Institut de Cancérologie et d'Immunogénétique, Hôpital Paul-Brousse, Villejuif [1], Hôpital Trousseau, Paris [2], Children's Cancer Research Foundation, Boston, MA [3], and Laboratory of Cell Biology, Cellular and Tumor Immunology Section, National Cancer Institute, Bethesda, MD [4]

Infectious pulmonary complications represent a major cause of death in immunosuppressed patients. Viruses have been frequently isolated from such patients. Table 1 lists the major various types of viruses that have been found. Herpes viruses are the most common agents. This group includes a) cytomegaloviruses (CMV) which have been repeatedly isolated from the lungs and from many tissues in patients under immunosuppressive therapy: b) Herpes zoster viruses which are responsible for varicella and zoster infections, and c) Herpes hominis.

Table 1. Viral agents most frequency isolated from patients under intensive or immunosuppressive chemotherapy

Herpes viruses:	
	Cytomegalovirus
	Varicella-zoster virus
	Herpes hominis
Respiratory viruses:	
	Adenoviruses
	Myxo- and paramyxo viruses:
	Respiratory syncytial virus
	Influenza and para-influenza viruses
	Measles virus
Other viruses:	
	Rubella virus
	Coxsackie and Echo viruses
	Hepatitis
	Reoviruses . . .

Respiratory viruses are also of great interest because viral pulmonary complications occur frequently in immunosuppressed patients. Adenoviruses, myxo- and paramyxoviruses, usually responsible for benign infections in children, have been also found in immunosuppressed patients. Other viruses have only rarely been incriminated.

We have given special attention to pulmonary complications (Fig. 1) such as those described by CLARYSSE *et al.* (1969) in patients treated with methotrexate (MTX). The Acute Leukemia Group B has reported the occurrence of pulmonary complications in 38/93 (41%) of their patients with acute lymphoid leukemia during maintenance of remission with intermittent MTX. It was suggested, but not proven, that the pulmonary disease represented an adverse allergic reaction to MTX therapy (Acute Leukemia Group B, 1969).

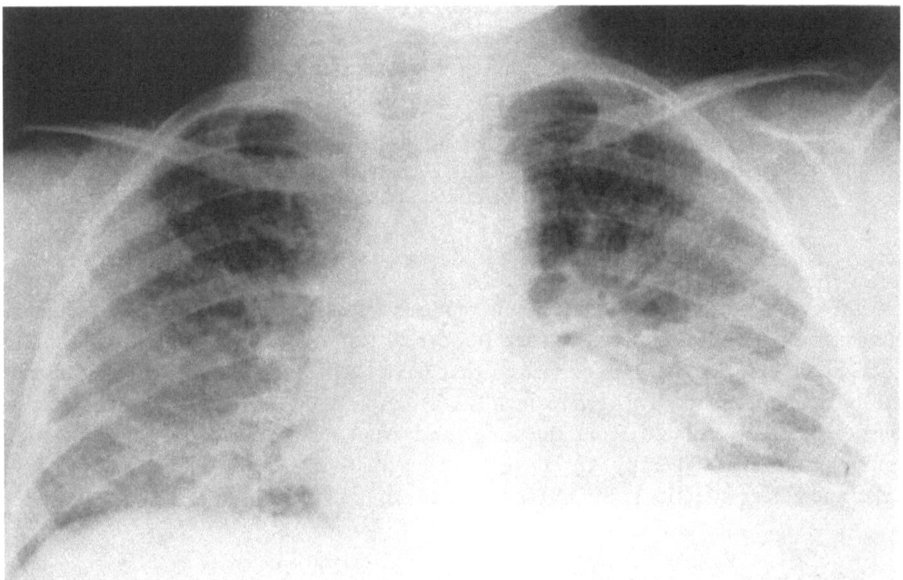

Fig. 1. Interstitial pneumonia in a patient treated with 6-mercaptopurine and methotrexate. Note the bilateral diffuse infiltration

We have designed a protocol (Table 2) to study systematically leukemic patients treated with the combination of 6 mercaptopurine (6 MP) and MTX. Patients received 5—15 mg/m² or methotrexate twice weekly and 50 to 70 mg/m² of 6 MP

Table 2. Protocol of virological studies of patients under intensive chemotherapy [a]

Before treatment, collect 5 ml of serum for determination of antibodies against 23 viruses.
During chemotherapy, each week a throat swab and 20 ml of urine were obtained and frozen at −70 °C within 30 minutes [b]. Serum (5 ml) was collected for serological studies.
After chemotherapy, serum (5 ml) was obtained every 2 months, when possible.
All sera from each patient were titrated simultaneously.

[a] Double blind studies.

[b] Samples were inoculated on stationary cultures of: Primary Green Monkey Kidney, $LLC\text{-}MK_2$ (Monkey Kidney), KB cells, Human diploid cells (WI 38).

daily according to the blood counts of the patients. Before treatment, 5 ml of serum was collected. During the administration of 6 MP-MTX, fresh throat and urine samples were collected weekly and inoculated on four types of cells. Simultaneously five ml of serum from each patient was collected and stored. When possible, sera were obtained after the phase of 6 MP-MTX.

Table 3 lists the 23 viruses included in the serological survey. It should be noticed that these studies were done on coded samples. At the present time, only 12 patients

Table 3. Serological studies

Virus	Technique used
Cytomegalovirus	Indirect hemagglutination
Herpes I	Indirect hemagglutination
Influenza A	Inhibition of hemagglutination
Influenza B	Inhibition of hemagglutination
Para-influenza 3	Inhibition of hemagglutination
Para-influenza 1	Complement fixation
Coxsackie B_1	Seroneutralization
Coxsackie B_2	Seroneutralization
Coxsackie B_3	Seroneutralization
Coxsackie B_4	Seroneutralization
Coxsackie B_5	Seroneutralization
Coxsackie B_6	Seroneutralization
Echeo 11	Seroneutralization
Rubella	Inhibition of hemagglutination
Measles	Inhibition of hemagglutination
Adenovirus	Complement fixation
Respiratory syncytial virus	Complement fixation
Mumps	Complement fixation
Varicella-Herpes Zoster	Complement fixation
Reovirus 1	Inhibition of hemagglutination
Reovirus 2	Inhibition of hemagglutination
Reovirus 3	Seroneutralization
Reovirus Laval [a]	Inhibition of hemagglutination

[a] Reovirus Laval has been isolated from a patient. It is closely related but not identical to Reovirus type 1.

have completed their study. Table 4 summarizes the data from these patients. Viruses could be isolated in 50% of patients with pulmonary complications whereas none were found in patients without pulmonary manifestations. Three reoviruses were isolated from throat swabs and one enterovirus from the urine. In the one case that came to autopsy, cytomegaloviruses were isolated from the lung.

Serologically, a seroconversion to parainfluenzae 3 and 1 was observed in one patient with pulmonary complications. The presence of IGM and IGG antibodies to these viruses and the absence of antibodies to parainfluenza 2 and to mumps virus suggest strongly a primary infection with parainfluenza 3 with a recall response to parainfluenza.

In another patient without pulmonary complication, antibodies to cytomegalovirus, herpes hominis type 1 and parainfluenza 3 rose simultaneously. This patient had low levels of antibodies to these viruses before any treatment. A transitory appearance of Forssman type antibodies against sheep red blood cells was also found in one patient with interstitial pneumonia. Patients from whom a reovirus was isolated remained serologically negative during the whole study.

Although these results are from only a limited number of patients, they suggest an infectious origin for these pulmonary complications. It is striking that in a double blind study, viruses were isolated in 50% of patients with pulmonary complications and none in the other group.

Table 4. Preliminary results

A. Virus isolation

	Patients with interstitial pneumonia	Patients without clinical or radiol. pneumonia
Urine	1/8	0/4
Throat	3/8	0/4

In 3 cases a reovirus type 1 was isolated from throat swabs.
In 1 case an enterovirus was isolated in the urine.
In 1 case a CMV was found at autopsy in the lung.

B. Serological study

	Patients with interstitial pneumonia	Patients without interstitial pneumonia
No serological modification	5	4
Increase in antibody titres	0	1
Serological conversion	2	0
Total	7	5

Reoviruses and enteroviruses are not considered to be endogenous viruses and they come most probably from exogenous sources. The unexpected isolation of 3 reoviruses type I suggests a horizontal transmission of these agents. How are these complications related to the immune status of patients treated with 6 MP-MTX? Our results do not suggest a humoral deficiency in patients with interstitial pneumonia. The titres of antibodies to viruses were comparable in patients without pneumonia and in patients before any treatment and two patients with pulmonary complications demonstrated their ability to make antibodies against a new antigen.

However, it is difficult to interpret the absence of seroconversion to reoviruses in patients from whom the agents were isolated. Possibilities include: low levels of virus, low antigenicity of viruses, and/or specific impairment of the primary humoral response. We need more data to answer these questions.

We have also investigated cell mediated immunity in these patients (Table 5). Patients reacted poorly to skin tests with recall antigens although two patients reacted to the first sensitizing applications of DNFB, a primary antigen. Lymphocytes showed a low reactivity to stimulation by PHA and PWM. No significant differences have been found between patients with and without pulmonary complications. Therefore, if immunosuppression can explain the severity of infection, it does not seem to account for the increased incidence of viral contaminations.

Table 5. Immune investigation in patients treated with a combination of mercaptopurine-methotrexate: correlations with pulmonary complications

	In vivo tests [a]				*In vitro* tests [b]		
	Tuberculine	Candidine	Mumps	DNFB	PHA	PWM	PPD
Patients without pulmonary complications	3/12	4/12	3/12	0/5	1/6	1/6	0/6
Patients with pulmonary complications	2/8	1/7	1/7	2[c]/10	1/3	0/3	0/3
Total	5/20	5/19	4/19	2/10	2/9	1/9	0/9

[a] N° of positive / N° of patients tested.
[b] N° of patients reacting normally / N° of patients tested.
[c] These 2 patients responded to the first application of DNFB.

In conclusion, these preliminary results demonstrate the high frequency of viral infections in immunosuppressed patients. Contamination of patients treated with 6 MP-MTX by viruses which generally have a low pathogenicity may provoke interstitial pneumonia with high efficacy. Other factors that we have not studied may be operative in these patients, such as: 1. the level of IGA in bronchial secretions, 2. the local production of interferon (Rytel and Balay, 1973), and 3. the activity of lung macrophages. Drastic prophylactic measures and the use of protected environments may eliminate or lower the risk of exogenous contamination.

The high incidence of pulmonary complications, the absence of predictive laboratory tests and the lack of antiviral drugs underline the problem of the toxic cost of the chemotherapy.

References

Acute leukemia group B: Acute lymphocytic leukemia in children: Maintenance therapy with methotrexate administered intermittently. J. Amer. med. Ass. **207**, 923 (1969).

Clarysse, A. M., Cathey, W. J., Cartwright, G. E. and Wintrobe, M. M.: Pulmonary disease complicating intermittent therapy with methotrexate. J. Amer. med. Ass. **209**, 1961 (1969).

Rytel, M. W., and Balay, J.: Impaired production of interferon in lymphocytes from immunosuppressed patients. J. infect. Dis. **127**, 445 (1973).

Role of Gnotobiotic Care in Chemotherapy of Acute Leukemia*

M. DIETRICH

Center for Internal Medicine and Pediatrics Division of Hematology, University of Ulm, Ulm

Introduction

Success in prolonging the survival of patients with acute leukemia (AL) is not attributed solely to application of chemotherapy but also to improved supportive care. Severe and often fatal infection remains a problem during induction of remission by chemotherapy. The difficulty in treating infections during the phase is due not only to the marked granulocytopenia resulting from bone marrow depletion but also to the fact that microorganisms normally present in the environment or the endogenous microflora may become pathogenic under these conditions. The aim of gnotobiotic care is to prevent infection by pathogens and potential pathogens.

We report our experience with patients aged 15—63 years diagnosed as having acute myelocytic leukemia (AML) or acute undifferentiated leukemia (AUL) and undergoing treatment with repeated courses of chemotherapy (including first, second and third relapses). The patients were either isolated, or isolated and decontaminated with nonabsorbable antibiotics.

Principle of Gnotobiotic Care

Patients in a normal environment are exposed to both environmental and endogenous microflora; isolated patients are at risk only from their own microbes; decontaminated patients in isolation are protected completely, once a "germ-free" state is achieved.

Reverse Isolation

The reverse isolation took place in a "Life Island" isolator and a completely tight plastic isolation system of our own construction (Ulm Isolator).

* Supported by the Deutsche Forschungsgemeinschaft, Sonderforschungsbereich 112, Zellsystemphysiologie.

This system gives the patient enough comfort to prevent the severe psychological reactions that may arise from restriction of daily activities and complete dependence on attending personnel (Fig. 1). The position of the bed inside the system can be regulated by a hydraulic system. A bellows in the plastic chamber can be extended to the wall of the room, thus doubling the space inside. All the electronic and hydraulic devices can be operated by the patient. The patient has enough space to take

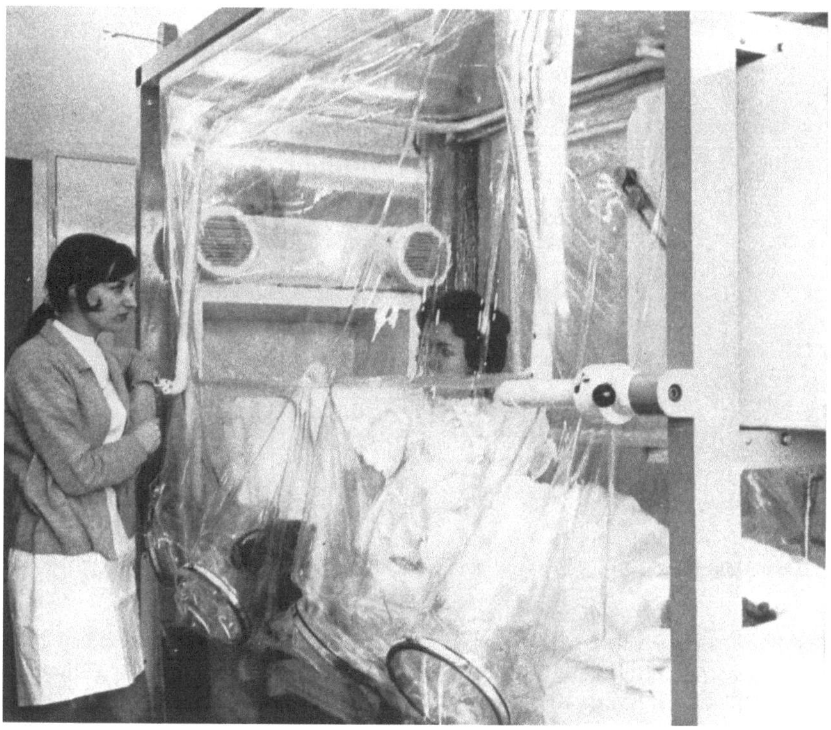

Fig. 1. Ulm isolated bed system

physical exercise. It must be emphasized that this is a completely airtight isolator in contrast to rooms with laminar air flow. We have found that with this system patients can be isolated for up to 4 months without severe psychological reactions. The work of the nurses is facilitated by the hydraulic aids, though it is more time-consuming than nursing on the open ward. However, we allot only one extra nurse to an isolated patient per 24 hours in addition to the regular nursing staff of the ward. While there are no real disadvantages in comparison with a laminar-air-flow room, we think there are some advantages. For instance, the barrier function of an isolator can be better controlled than in a room with unidirectional airflow. Such reported incidents as insects passing the isolation barrier, children leaving isolation, and relatives handing an unsterile birthday cake into the room make the laminar-air-flow room a less controllable isolation device.

Decontamination

Decontamination from microflora is achieved by surface disinfection and non-absorbable antibiotics, application of local antibiotics to the orifices of the body, and treatment of existing infections by systemic antibiotics (Fig. 2).

In accordance with reports in the literature, our experience shows that in adults with AL most of the stool specimens are bacteriologically negative, but cultures of skin swabs less so. Oral washings and mouth swabs are rarely without microbial growth. In our series only 7% did not show any growth.

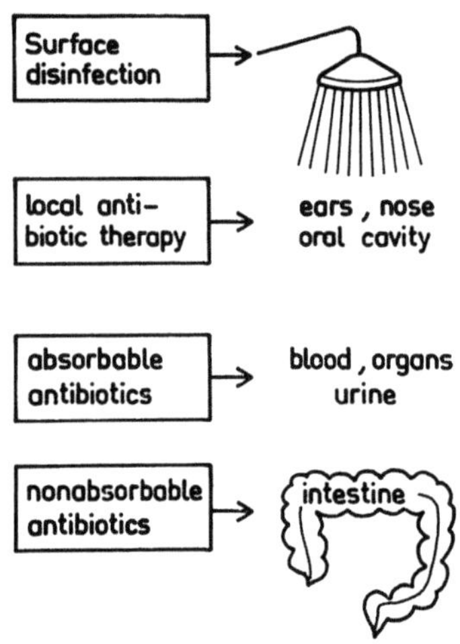

Fig. 2. Decontamination procedures by antibiotic treatment and use of Disinfecting agents

From the use of the combination of nonabsorbable antimicrobial agents. *N*eomycin sulfate, *B*acitracin sulfate, *N*ystatin and *P*olymycin B we saw a number of side-effects, both negative and positive. Nausea may occur, loss of appetite and allergies. For example d-xylose absorption is decreased markedly during the decontamination phase. It is not clear how the decontamination process may affect cytostatic therapy, especially, when oral drugs are used. There could be some pharmacodynamic interaction.

Hemostatic studies were compared in patients with and without decontamination therapy, grouped by different platelet counts. The parameter used was the maximal elasticity of the thrombus formation. The complete data are published elsewhere (DIETRICH *et al.*, 1973). The results indicate that decontaminated patients have better thrombus formation. At the present time we do not know which factor causes this phenomenon.

Efficiency of Gnotobiotic Care

To evaluate the efficiency of gnotobiotic treatment of these patients, we may count the percentage of remissions. The data were obtained in retrospect for 30 patients who, on the first sign of disease or on further relapses, were isolated only, or both isolated and decontaminated. No comparison was made with patients in the open ward because this was not a randomized study. There was complete remission in 57% of the patients, and 83% achieved complete or partial remission; 80% of the patients survived for 30 days after the period of treatment was terminated. This result is comparable to the data in the literature. Bodey *et al.* found 60% complete remission in a retrospective study, Levine *et al.* recently reported a 45% rate of remission in a prospective study. Both teams stated that there was no significant difference between the remission rate of patients in the open ward and those in the isolation-decontamination program. In our observation, failure to achieve remission could not be correlated with age, with degree of granulocytopenia, nor with the number of days with fever above 38 °C (Figs. 3—5). This suggests that the remission rate cannot be affected in any way by the use of gnotobiotic care.

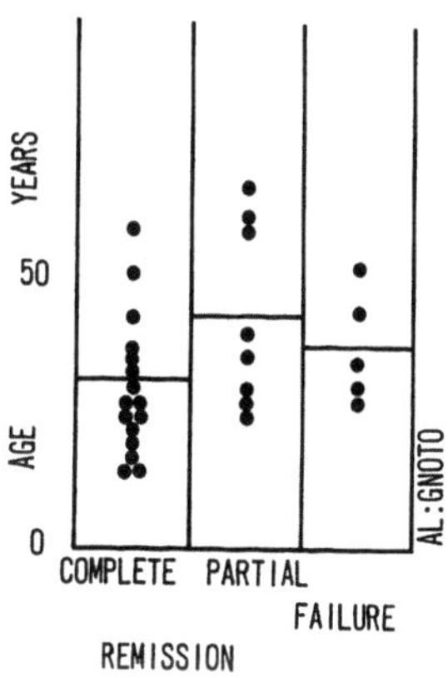

Fig. 3

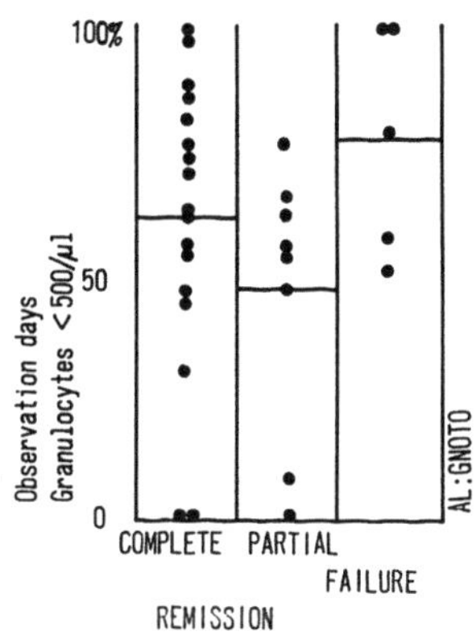

Fig. 4

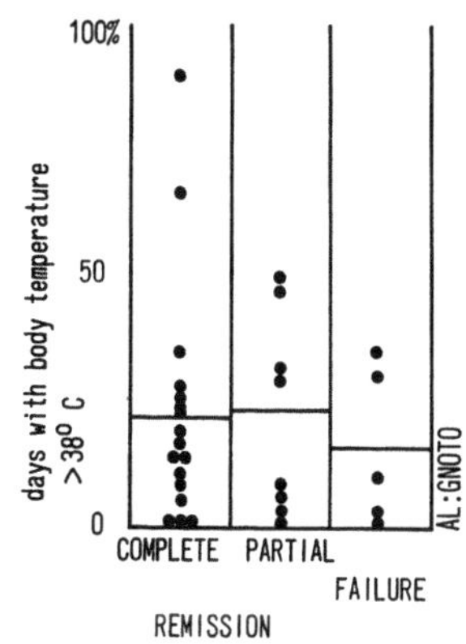

Fig. 5

Fig. 3. Age of isolated patients with complete remission, partial remission or failure (mean values)

Fig. 4. Observation days on which granulocyte count was below 500/μl (mean values)

Fig. 5. Percentage of observation days on which the body temperature of isolated patients was above 38 °C (measured three times daily)

Are there any other benefits for the patients? Levine *et al.* reported that about one quarter of the patients in the open ward died from infections during the induction therapy phase but none died in the isolation-decontamination program. The results of the retrospective study of Bodey *et al.* indicate a significantly longer duration of remission in the decontaminated and isolated patients. However, this beneficial effect could perhaps be attributed to the use of larger doses of cytostatic drugs.

As reported by Levine *et al.*, we observed that isolated patients did not succumb to severe respiratory infections, which suggests that airbone infection can be prevented by isolation (Table 1).

On evaluating the course of individual patients randomized one or more times to different treatment groups during repeated trials of induction of remission, we

Table 1. Incidence of severe respiratory infection in patients receiving different types of care

Group	Treatment cycles	Severe respiratory infection
A (reverse isolation and decontamination)	9	None
B (reverse isolation)	14	None
C	13	5

Group A — isolation + decontamination
Group B — isolation
Group C — open ward

found an interesting but very preliminary observation (Table 2). Patients between 16 and 60 years of age were randomized to group A (isolation and decontamination), group B (isolation only) and group C (treatment in the open ward). A patient who was treated one or more times in group A or group B was counted in group A or B, respectively, even if he was treated also in the open ward at other treatment periods. Those in group C were treated exclusively in the open ward. The period of observation included at least six months after chemotherapy for the induction of remission was terminated. Patients treated in groups A and B tended to survive for longer. This could be understood as longer duration of single remissions, or it could

Table 2. Survival of patients receiving different types of care

Group	A	B	C
Patients	8	11	8
CR (several treatments)	10	17	7
Mean survival	50	59	29
Median survival (weeks)	52 (8—100)	49 (18—96)	20 (2—97)
Still living	5	5	2

Group A — isolation + decontamination
Group B — isolation
Group C — open ward

be that these patients have fewer complications due to infection and therefore tolerate more chemotherapeutic trials. There are a number of factors involved, so that any conclusion is very difficult and has to be taken with caution. However, it might be worthwhile to follow up further observations.

References

Dietrich, M., Rasche, H., Rommel, K., Hochapfel, G.: Antimicrobial therapy as a part of the decontamination procedures for patients with acute leukemia. Europ. J. Cancer **9**, 443 (1973).

Bodey, G. P., Gehan, E. A., Freireich, E. J. *et al.*: Protected environment-prophylactic antibiotic program in the chemotherapy of acute leukemia. J. Amer. med. Sci. **262**, 138 (1971).

Levine, A. S., Siegel, S. E., Schreiber, A. D. *et al.*: Protected environments and prophylactic antibiotics. New Engl. J. Med. **288**, 10, 477 (1973).

Mathé, G. (ed.): Aseptic environments and cancer treatment. In Recent Results in Cancer Research. Vol. 29. Springer: Berlin, Heidelberg, New York 1970.

White Blood Cell Transfusions in Leukemic Patients with Severe Infections

A. Bussel, M. Benbunan, M. Weil, J. Reviron, C. Jacquillat, M. Boiron, and J. Bernard

Service du Professeur Jean Bernard, Institut de Recherches sur les Maladies du Sang et les Leucémies, Hôpital Saint-Louis, Paris

Introduction

Infection is the most common complication in acute leukemia; management of infections has a direct influence on the results of chemotherapy, especially in acute granulocytic leukemia. We report here our experience with white blood cell (WBC) transfusions.

As shown in Table 1, a total of 1563 transfusions have been done, 1497 from 229 donors with chronic myelocytic leukemia (CML) and 66 from 60 normal donors; the total number of recipients was 789. Patients who received transfusions of normal WBC represent a homogeneous group, treated by the same protocol.

Table 1. Number of WBC transfusions, of recipients, of donors and dose of granulocytes

Number of WBC transfusions		Number of recipients	Number of donors	Amount of transfused granulocytes
CML	1497	748	229	1×10^{11}/sqm
Normal	66	41	60	4.51×10^{10} average
Total	1563	789	289	

Transfusions From CML Donors

Granulocyte transfusions from CML donors have been used with increasing frequency since this source of cells was first suggested by Morse (1961, 1966). The method used in the present study was the classic plasmaphoresis technique with addition of modified fluid gelatin (MFG) and sedimentation. Prior to transfusion, the leukocytes are concentrated at low speed (180 g for 13 min). The calculated dose to be transfused is 1.0×10^{11} cells per m^2 body area of the recipient. We found red cell contamination to be less than 1% (hematocit).

Table 2 shows the tests performed on the donor; clinical examination excluded contraindications such as cardiovascular disease. The WBC count was always more than 100,000/mm³ and bone marrow aspiration and biopsy should exclude the possibility of acute transformation of CML. ABO Rh compatibility is not necessary with such low red cell contamination. If hemolysins were present in the donor, the buffy coat was washed in saline. Alloantibodies against leukocytes and red blood cells were looked for; direct crossmatching between donor's cells and recipients' serum had to be negative by the agglutination technique. Serological examinations were made to detect any recent infection such as syphilis, hepatitis, toxoplasmosis, or cytomegalovirus.

Table 2. Tests on donors with CML

— Clinical exam.	
— Hematological exam.	
	hemogram: W.B.C > 100 000/mm³
	bone marrow aspiration
	bone marrow biopsy
— Immuno hematol exam.	
	ABO Rh typing
	red cells alloantibodies and hemolysines res.
	platelets allo antibodies res.
— Serological exam.	
	B.W.
	Australia
	Anticytomegalovirus (C.M.V.) antibodies titration
	Antitoxoplasmosis antibodies titration

Table 3 shows the diagnoses in the recipients. We limit our analysis to 753 severe infections observed in 661 patients with acute leukemias who received 1332 transfusions.

Table 3. Analysis of recipients of WBC transfusions

	No. of patients	Total no. of	Cases of
Acute leukemia and diffuse LBS	661	1332	753
Other hematol. diseases	54	132	63
Miscellaneous	33	33	33
Total	748	1497	849

Table 4 reports the status of the 661 patients prior to transfusion. All had severe infections, focal sepsis, septicemia, or fever. Most had no circulating granulocytes and depleted bone marrow.

Table 4. Symptoms of recipients before WBC transfusions (753 severe infections)

Clinical	fever	97
	focal infections	557
	septicemia	278
Blood	granulocytes 0	644
	granulocytes $< 50/mm^3$	75
	granulocytes $50 < \quad < 1000/mm^3$	34
Bone marrow	acellular	398
	hypocellular and blastic	158
	blastic	128
	showing some regener.	69

Table 5. Relation between recovery of CML leucocytes after transfusion and clinical results

Recipients WBC/mm^3 after transfusion	No. of infections	Fall in temp.	Persistent fever
$\leqq 1000$	286	77 (27%)	209 (73%)
> 1000	467	387 (83%)	80 (17%)
Total	753	464 (62%)	289 (38%)

Table 6. Relation between patients age and diagnosis and results of WBC transfusion (753 infections)

Age	Diagnosis	No. of infections	Success	Percent
Adults	AML	338	189	56%
	ALL LBS	86	50	58%
Children	AML	82	66	81%
	ALL LBS	247	161	70%

Table 7. Relation between ABO Rh compatibility and results of CML, WBC transfusions (753 infections)

ABO Rh compatibility	Success	Failure
–	285 (61%)	181 (29%)
+	180 (63%)	107 (27%)
	465	288

The criteria of the efficacy of WBC transfusion were fall in temperature within 48 hours with cure of the infection. As shown in Table 5, temperature fell in 464 patients (62%). The frequency of temperature fall was related to the post-transfusion granulocyte count: 387 patients (83%) who became afebrile had more than 1000 circulating granulocytes/mm^3 18 hours after the completion of transfusion. As can be seen in Table 6, results are significantly better in children than in adults but there is no difference between results observed in ALL and in AML.

The effect of red blood cells groups on the response to WBC transfusions is analysed on Table 7. AB0 incompatibility between donor red cells and recipient's plasma does not seem to influence clinical outcome. Survival of transfused cells was studied previously (Bussel *et al.*, 1971) and failed to demonstrate any role of AB0 group antigens in granulocyte recovery 18 hours after transfusion.

The complications observed with transfusions from CML donors are listed in Table 8. Of the 7% of patients who had chills, most had a poor recovery of transfused cells; these effects may be related to leukocyte antibodies undetected by leukoagglutination. No relation was found with AB0-group incompatibility.

Circulating hyperbasophilic cells were observed during the first week in 3% of cases. A mixed lymphocyte reaction could be evoked *in vivo*, as reported after blood transfusions (Schechter *et al.*, 1972); no infection was detected in these cases. A mononucleosis-like syndrome was observed in 2% of cases between weeks 4 and 6; in 12 of these 27 patients cytomegalovirus infections was indicated by an increase of cytomegalovirus complement-fixing antibodies. A serological study of these pa-

Table 8. Complications of 1332 WBC transfusions from CML donors to 661 patients with AL

Minor	Cases	%	Major	Cases	%
Chills	99	7	Shock	4	0.3
Early circulating hyperbasophilic cells (1st week)	40	3	Respiratory failure	10	0.7
			Renal failure	15	1
Mononucleosis syndrome	27 [a]	2	GVH reaction	6 to 8 grafts	0.4

[a] 12 of the 27 patients had cytomegalovirus infection.

tients' donors failed to detect evidence of cytomegalovirus infection; however, asymptomatic viremia has been demonstrated in normal donors (Diost *et al.*, 1969), and WBC transfusions may represent a common origin for cytomegalovirus infection in leukemia patients.

Respiratory failure was observed mainly in patients with severe pulmonary infections. In view of the possibility of tissue sequestration of WBC, particularly in the lungs, it would seem hazardous to transfuse a large mass of WBC into patients with minimal respiratory function; if transfusion is necessary, dose and rate of injection should be low.

Progressive renal failure with anuria was observed in 15 recipients. All of them received repeated daily transfusions without clinical effect. Renal failure was unrelated to red cell AB0 group; no anti-leukocyte antibodies were detected in either the recipients' or the donors' serum; however, it may be postulated that leukocyte incompatibility plays a role in renal disease.

Severe GVH reactions were observed in 5 patients with 8 proven grafts (Table 9). Similar manifestations of secondary disease after CML leukocyte transfusion have been reported in detail by MATHÉ *et al.* To prevent development of a secondary syndrome, buffy coats are now X-irradiated with 1000 rads before infusion (GRAW, *et al.*, 1970).

Table 9. Analysis of cases of GVH after transfusions of WBC from CML donors (6/1332)

Case	Infused granul./kg	AB0 Rh compatibility	Age years	Stage of disease	Prior chemotherapy	Tests of grafts			GVH
						Phl	Double AB0 pp.	Donors HLA type	
O. 1	3.5×10^9	+	55	AML 1st relapse	Ara-C 22 050 RP	+	0	0	+ Death
L. 2	2.2×10^9	–	24	AML 1st attack	DNR+Asp.+ Ara-C+cyclo.	+	0	0	+ Death
M. 3	6×10^9	–	4	ALL 1st relapse	DNR+Asp. Ara-C+cyclo.	–	–	+	+ Death
N. 4	11×10^9	+	69	AML 1st attack	0	+	–	+	+ Death
V. 5	6×10^9	–	50	AML + Hodgkin	22 050 RP	+	–	–	+ Death
Q. 6	2.2×10^9	–	47	AML relapse	DNR+ Asp.	+	0	0	+ Death

Transfusions of Granulocytes From Normal Donors

Transfusions of normal leukocytes from a single donor have become practical with the introduction of the continuous-flow blood cell separator (GRAW *et al.*, 1971, 1972).

Heparin was used as anticoagulant. Yield of granulocytes was increased by administering intravenous hydrocortisone to the donor (100 mg, 150 min before leukophoresis; 50 mg, 20 min prior to commencement; 75 mg during separation). The addition of macromolecular compounds such as MFG or hydroxyethylstarch (McCREDIE *et al.*, 1971) to increase red cell rouleaux formation can greatly augment granulocyte recovery: 1000 ml of MFG was introduced into the input line of the blood cell separator. As reported (BENBUNAN *et al.*, 1973), 200 mg of heparin was added in the first 500 ml of MFG. An average of 11.9 l of whole blood was processed in 5 hours.

The volume of buffy coat was 500 ml and red-cell contamination about 30% (hematocrit). The buffy coat red cells were returned to the donor.

All normal donors were typed for red cell compatibility with the recipient; direct cross-matching should be negative with both the agglutination and the lymphocytotoxicity technique.

As can be seen from Table 10, the average number of leukocytes collected was 48×10^9 (94% of granulocytes), and of granulocytes per liter of whole blood processed 3.8×10^9.

Table 10. Machine run data and results

Runs	Anticoagulant	Donor's stimulation	Macro-molecular compound	WBC flow rate ML / MN	RPM centrifugation
	Heparin	Hydrocortisone	MFG	1.5—2	400
66	Volume processed per liter	Buffy coat volume (ML)	RBC contamination (hematocrit)	Total WBC collected per liter	Granulocytes per liter
	11.9	500	30%	4 10^9	3,8 10^9

[a] Modified fluid gelatin.

The clinical and hematological status of the recipients prior to WBC transfusion are summarized in Table 11. All patients had severe infections and had received a combination of broad-spectrum antibiotics without result.

Table 11. Symptoms of recipients before normal WBC transfusions (44 severe infections)

Fever		39
Septicemia		21
Focal infections		27
Blood granulocytes/mm^3	$= 0$	22
	$\leqq 500$	17
	> 500	5

Table 12. Relation between dose of normal WBC and WBC increment in recipient

Dose	Recipients WBC after transfusions $\geqq$ 1000/mm	Recipients WBC after transfusions $<$ 1000/mm
$\geqq 5 \times 10^{10}$/sqm	19 (95%)	1 (5%)
$< 5 \times 10^{10}$/sqm	17 (37%)	29 (63%)

Transfusion efficiency was estimated from the recipient's clinical course during the 24 hours following leukocyte transfusion. There was a strong correlation between dose and granulocyte increment: if the dose was equal to or greater than $5 \times 10^{10}/m^2$, 96% of patients had more than $1000/mm^3$ granulocytes after transfusion (Table 12). There was also a strong correlation between increase of WBC and clinical results; for instance, improvement was noted in 97% of patients with more than $1000/mm^3$ whereas the success rate was only 43% in patients with granulocyte count below $1000/mm^3$ (Table 13).

No side-effects were observed after normal leukocyte transfusions.

Table 13. Relation between granulocyte increment in recipients and clinical results after normal WBC transfusions

Recipients' granulocytes (per mm 3)	Success	Failure
≥ 1000	35 (97%)	1 (3%)
< 1000	13 (43%)	17 (57%)

Conclusion

We conclude that WBC from CML donors should be given only to patients with malignancy; AB0 and Rh compatibility is not important. The usual dose given was 1×10^{11} granulocytes/m^2.

Normal granulocytes may be given to all granulopenic patients. Careful choice of donors is necessary to avoid incompatibility. The usual yield was 5×10^{10} cells; this quantity represents the effective dose per square meter; hence transfusions need to be repeated in adults whereas one transfusion may be sufficient in children.

References

Benbunan, M., Bussel, A., Reviron, J., Boiron, M., Bernard, J.: Les transfusions de granulocytes normaux pré le vés sur séparateur de cellules. Résultats techniques et cliniques. Nouv. Rev. franç. hémat. **13**, 469 (1973).

Bussel, A., Benbunan, M., Tanzer, J., Boiron, M.: Transfusions de leucocytes au cours des aplasies après chimiothérapie antileucémique. Ed. Masson. Actual. Hémat. **5**, 169 (1971).

Diost, P., Moldovan, E., Tomescu, N.: Latent cytomegalovirus infection in blood donors. Brit. med. J. **1969 IV**, 600.

Graw, R. G., Buckner, C. D., Whang-Peng, J. S., Leventhal, B. C., Kruger, G., Berard, C., Henderson, E. S.: Complication of bone marrow transplantation: graft-versus-host disease resulting from chronic myelogenous leukemia leucocyte transfusion. Lancet **1790 II**, 338.

Graw, R. G., Herzig, G. P., Eisel, R. S., Perry, S.: Leukocyte and platelet collection from normal donors with the continuous flow blood cell separator. Transfusion **11**, 94 (1971).

Graw, R. G. Jr., Herzig, G. P., Perry, S., Henderson, E. S.: Normal granulocyte transfusion therapy. Treatment of septicemia due to Gram negative bacteria. New. Engl. J. Med. **287**, 367 (1972).

McCredie, K. B., Freireich, E. J.: Increased granulocyte collection from normal donors with increased granulocyte recovery following transfusion. Proc. Amer. Ass. Cancer Res. **12,** 58 (1971) (abstract n° 232).

Morse, E. E., Bronson, W., Carbone, P. P., Freireich, E. J.: Effectiveness of granulocyte transfusion from donors with chronic myelocytic leukemia to patients with leukopenia. Clin. Res. **9,** 332 (1961).

Morse, E. E., Freireich, E. J., Carbone, P. P., Bronson, W., Frei, E.: The transfusion of leukocytes from donors with chronic myelocytic leukemia to patients with leukopenia. Transfusion **6,** 183 (1966).

Schechter, G., Soehnlen, F., McFarland, W.: Lymphocyte response to blood transfusion in man. New. Engl. J. Med. **287,** 1169 (1972).

Schwarzenberg, L., Mathé, G., DeGrouchy, J., DeNava, C., Devries, M. S., Amiel, S. L., Cattan, A., Schneider, M., Schlumberger, J. R.: White blood cell transfusion. Israel J. Med. Sci. **1,** 925 (1965).

Efficacy of Platelet Transfusions from HL-A Compatible Unrelated Donors to Alloimmunized Patients*

H.-P. LOHRMANN, M. I. BULL, J. A. DECTER, R. A. YANKEE, and R. G. GRAW, JR.

National Cancer Institute, National Institutes of Health, Bethesda, MD

Transfusion support of thrombocytopenic patients with platelet concentrates has considerably reduced the incidence of life-threatening bleeding complications (DJERASSI *et al.*, 1963; ALVARADO *et al.*, 1965; FREIREICH, 1966; HAN *et al.*, 1966; CAVINS *et al.*, 1968). However, alloimmunization to random donor platelet antigens with resultant refractoriness to platelet transfusions regularly develops in polytransfused patients, which makes effective long-term platelet support difficult (BALDINI *et al.*, 1961; SHULMAN, 1966; GRUMET and YANKEE, 1970). In these situations, platelets obtained from siblings genotypically identical for their lymphocyte HL-A antigens resulted in post transfusion increments normally found only in non alloimmunized individuals (GRUMET and YANKEE, 1970; YANKEE *et al.*, 1969). This has been interpreted as evidence that the most important antigenic determinants for platelet compatibility are represented by or closely linked to the HL-A locus (the genetic locus coding for the major human transplantation antigen system). Although the few defined platelet-specific non-HL-A antigens may lead to the development of alloantibodies, they are an uncommon cause of alloimmunization (SVEJGAARD, 1969; ADNER *et al.*, 1969) since these antigens are shared by a high percentage of the population (SHULMAN *et al.*, 1964; DAUSSET and TANGUN, 1965).

YANKEE *et al.* (1973) transfused three selected thrombocytopenic alloimmunized patients with platelets obtained from HL-A compatible unrelated donors. Their report indicated that matching of donor and recipient by lymphocyte HL-A types could help to overcome a major problem in selecting platelet donors by platelet antigens: Alloimmunized patients requiring platelet support are often markedly thrombocytopenic, making determination of their platelet surface antigens technically difficult. The lack of sensitive and widely available antisera for defining platelet antigens further limits the utility of platelet typing (SVEJGAARD, 1969).

The present study was undertaken in order to further evaluate in a larger population of unselected alloimmunized patients the usefulness of selecting unrelated platelet donors by their lymphocyte HL-A antigens.

---

* This work has been published in more detail in the Annals of Internal Medicine, January 1974.

Methods and Patients

Lymphocyte HL-A typing was performed by Dr. Paul I. Terasaki, University of California, Los Angeles, using the micro-lymphocytotoxicity technique (MITTAL *et al.*, 1968). A computer program (developed by RAY MICKEY, Ph. D., Department of Biomathematics, University of California, Los Angeles) was used to search a file, which currently contains 3,000 HL-A typed normal donors, for HL-A compatibility with a particular patient. The donors were HL-A retyped at the first platelet donation to confirm their HL-A type.

HL-A compatibility was considered to exist when none of the identified donor antigens were different from those of the recipient. The classification of HL-A compatibilities used in this context is as follows:

A-match: HL-A phenotype identity of donor and recipient of all defined antigens on first and second sublocus.

B-match: All the donor's HL-A antigens are present in the recipient's phenotype; however, the donor does not possess all the recipient's HL-A antigens. B-1 and B-2-match are subclassifications of the B-group and indicate that 1 or 2 antigens defined in the recipient could not be detected in the donor.

Mismatch: The donor possesses HL-A antigen(s) that are not found in the recipient. Due to the extreme polymorphism of the HL-A system, random donor platelets can be considered to be mismatched.

(Examples of the classification used: Recipient phenotype 1,2,8,12; A-matched donor 1,2,8,12; B-1-matched donor 1,2,12 or 1,8,12 etc.; B-2-matched donor 1,12 or 2,12 etc.; mismatched donor 1,2,7,12).

HL-A compatible donors found on the computer file were selected for platelet donations only on the basis of their availability. Attempts were made to use as many different donors for a particular patient as possible. Incompatibility of the donors in the ABO system was disregarded in the selection process.

Platelets from 2—4 units of whole blood (1 unit = 500 ml) were collected by the "split-ACD" technique (CHAPPELL, 1966); the combined platelet concentrates were transfused within 4 hours after procurement. Visual platelet counts (BRECHER and CRONKITE, 1950) on the recipients were done on the morning of the platelet transfusion and, whenever possible, both 1 and 20 hours after its completion. The post transfusion increments (platelet count post transfusion, minus platelet count prior to transfusion) were corrected according to the formula (YANKEE *et al.*, 1969):

$$\begin{array}{l}\text{Corrected}\\ \text{transfusion}\\ \text{increment}\end{array} = \frac{\text{Transfusion increment (per cu mm) X BSA (m2)}}{\text{Number of units transfused}}$$

The formula corrects the actually observed post transfusion platelet increments for the number of units given, and for weight and height (SENDROY and CECCHINI, 1954) of the recipient. It thus allows to compare responses to platelet transfusions in different individuals.

Thrombocytopenia in the patients included in this study was a result of aplastic anemia, leukemia or chemotherapy of various malignancies. Patients were considered alloimmunized or refractory when in the absence of sepsis, splenomegaly or disseminated intravascular coagulation platelets obtained from different mismatched donors repeatedly resulted in corrected 20 hour post transfusion increments of $<$2500/cmm X BSA / unit (YANKEE *et al.*, 1969). All throbocytopenic alloimmunized patients requiring platelet support were included in the study provided HL-A compatible donors were available.

Transfusions of platelets to patients with sepsis, disseminated intravascular coagulation and splenomegaly are not reported, since these conditions may alter the response to platelet transfusions even in the absence of alloimmunization. When a donor was used repeatedly for a particular patient due to consistently good transfusion responses, the increments to only the first 2 transfusions were averaged for comparison with other donor-recipient pairs. This, rather than including every given transfusion separately, was done as not to bias the data towards the favorable responses. Since effective platelet support will result only when long-lasting platelet increments are obtained following a platelet transfusion, the 20 hour rather than the 1 hour post transfusion platelet increments are used to compare platelet transfusions from HL-A compatible, and from mismatched donors.

The titres of the homologous isoagglutinins anti-A and anti-B were determined in serum samples obtained from the recipients immediately prior to platelet transfusions from an AB0-incompatible platelet donor, and stored at -70 degrees. The assay was performed by Mary H. McGinniss, NIH, Clinical Center, Blood Bank, with standard blood bank techniques using serial saline dilutions of the sera to be tested.

Results and Discussion

15 alloimmunized patients refractory to random donor platelets were supported with platelets from unrelated donors who were compatible for their lymphocyte HL-A types. As Table 1 shows, 18 HL-A identical donors were used for 8 patients on 54 occasions, 29 B-1-matched donors were plateletpheresed for 10 patients on 104

Table 1. Platelet transfusions from HL-A compatible donors to alloimmunized patients

Patients in study	15		
Match grade [a]	A-match	B-1-match	B-2-match
Number of patients	8	10	8
Number of donors	18	29	25
Number of transfusions	54	104	48

[a] For explanation, see text.

occasions, and 25 B-2-matched donors were used for 8 patients on 48 occasions. The time of support with HL-A matched platelets varied from 1—48 weeks. None of the 15 patients included in this study died of hemorrhage; 6 of them succumbed to other complications of their underlying disease. 9 patients are alive at present, and continue to be supported with platelets from the original HL-A compatible unrelated donors. No refractoriness to these donors' platelets has developed.

Fig. 1 depicts the corrected 20 hour post transfusion increments in the various donor-recipient pairs, arranged by the degree of HL-A compatibility. In Table 2, the corrected 1 hour and 20 hour post transfusion platelet increments (Increment X m2 / unit) after platelet transfusions from HL-A compatible, and from HL-A Mismatched donors are statistically analysed.

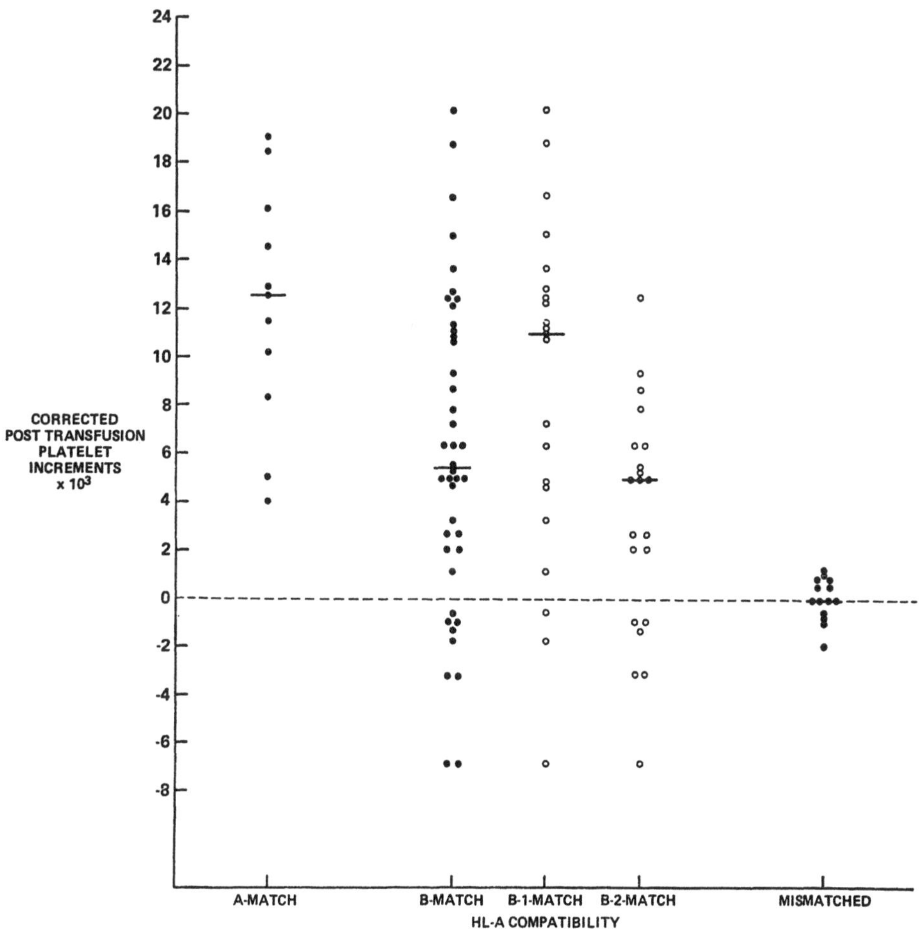

Fig. 1. Corrected 20 hours post transfusion platelet increments (Increments X m2 / unit) following HL-A compatible, and HL-A mismatched platelet transfusions in alloimmunized patients. Each closed circle represents one single donor-recipient pair. Donor-recipient pairs of the B-group have been subdivided into B-1 and B-2-matches, as shown by open circles. The horizontal lines indicate the medians. See text for the classification of HL-A compatibilities

As can be seen from Fig. 1 and Table 2, A-matched donors gave high transfusion increments, while transfusions from mismatched donors failed to increase the platelet count. B-matched donors gave intermediate platelet increments. However, when the latter group is analysed by the number of excess HL-A antigens in the recipient, remarkable differences exist:

Taking the lowest 20 hour post transfusion platelet increment observed in A-matched donor-recipient pairs as a limit (i. e., 4000 X m2/unit), it can be seen from Fig. 1 that 27/42 of the B-donors gave high platelet increments, whereas 15/42 gave poor or no increments. The latter are responsible for the overall reduced increments in the B-group and, since they are predominantly represented by B-2-matched donors (10/15), for the poor increments in this subgroup.

Table 2. Comparison of transfusion responses as related to HL-A compatibility

Degree of HL-A compatibility [a]		Median [b]	p-value [c]	
1 hour post transfusion				
A-match	(17) [d]	15 000	A vs. B-1 :	N.S. [e]
			A vs. B-2 :	< 0.001
B-match	(48)	11 200		
B-1-match	(25)	14 700	B-1 vs. B-2 :	< 0.001
B-2-match	(23)	6 300		
20 hours post transfusion				
A-match	(11)	12 500	A vs. B-1 :	N.S.
			A vs. B-2 :	< 0.001
			A vs. mismatch :	< 0.001
B-match	(42)	5 300		
B-1-match	(21)	10 900	B-1 vs. B-2 :	< 0.005
			B-1 vs. mismatch :	< 0.001
B-2-match	(21)	4 800	B-2 vs. mismatch :	< 0.001
Mismatch	(30)	0		

[a] For explanation, see text.
[b] Calculated from the corrected increments (Increments X m2 / unit).
[c] As determined by the Wilcoxon rank sum test.
[d] Numbers in brackets indicate numbers of evaluable donor-recipient pairs; the number of evaluated pairs differ at 1 and 20 hours post transfusion, since platelet counts at both times were not done in all recipients.
[e] N.S. = Not significant.

The lower the number of defined HL-A specificities in an individual is, the more likely the result of the HL-A typing is incomplete. A higher percentage of B-2-donors than B-1-donors may than be expected to be typed incompletely, and will therefore be mismatched with their respective recipient. Serologically not identified HL-A specificities are therefore most likely to account for the differences between the 2 subgroups.

Our data confirm the preliminary data by YANKEE *et al.* (1973) that well phenotyped HL-A compatible unrelated donors can be used for effective long-term platelet support of alloimmunized patients. A stepwise decrease in the post transfusion platelet increments exists from HL-A identical to B-1-matched to B-2-matched to mismatched donor-recipient pairs (Fig. 1). This close correlation between the degree of HL-A compatibility and the post transfusion platelet increments in a large number of unrelated donor-recipient pairs establishes HL-A antigens as the most important antigens of human blood platelets. This does not exclude the possibility that in a few patients antibodies against platelet-specific antigens may develop, and then abolish transfusion responses even to HL-A identical platelet transfusions; this was not observed in our series.

Reports by THORSBY *et al.* (1972) and DAUSSET *et al.* (1970), and our own observations (YANKEE *et al.*, 1971) indicate that HL-A 12 may not be represented on platelets of some individuals carrying this antigen on their lymphocytes. Thus, it may be that donors mismatched for certain lymphocyte antigens may be found to be HL-A compatible for platelet transfusion purposes. Since at the present time our knowledge of the distribution of HL-A antigens on different blood cells is limited, selection of unrelated platelet donors for alloimmunized patients by compatibility for their lymphocyte HL-A antigens seems to be the only practical approach.

11 donors carried an incompatible B-antigen, and 8 an incompatible A-antigen on their red cells. Within the different groups of donor-recipient HL-A compatibility (A, B-1, B-2), there were no significant differences in the post transfusion platelet increments between AB0 compatible and incompatible donors. This is valid when the AB0-incompatible donors are considered as a single group, or when donors incompatible for A or B are evaluated separately.

From results of *in vitro* experiments, there is controversy as to whether or not the red blood cell antigens A and B are present on platelets (for ref., see SVEJGAARD, 1969). Our observations lend support to the concept that there is no A or B substance present on platelets. Our results confirm data reported by SHULMAN (1966) and FREIREICH *et al.* (1963); in contrast, ASTER (1965) and PFISTERER *et al.* (1968) reported decreased recoveries but normal intravascular survival of platelets from AB0-incompatible donors. These authors explained their findings with a possible "innocent bystander" involvement of the transfused platelets in a reaction against simultaneously transfused incompatible red cells, rather than recognition of AB-antigen on the platelet surface. The differences in the post transfusion responses to AB0 incompatible platelets in the former reports and in the present study may possibly be explained by lower red blood cell contamination in our platelet concentrates: our collection process results in a total red cell contamination of 0.5 ml/4 units.

The general application of HL-A matched platelet transfusions is presently limited to large medical centers possessing HL-A typing laboratories, computer assistance and financial support. Whether it is necessary or even feasible to transfuse a patient requiring long-term support with HL-A matched platelets from the onset of thrombocytopenia remains to be examined. However, once a patient is alloimmunized to random donor platelets, efforts should be made to obtain platelets from HL-A matched donors. The data presented in this study indicate that platelets from both A-matched and B-1-matched donors are likely to give normal post transfusion increments in alloimmunized patients, whereas transfusions from B-2-matched donors will only occasionally result in such increments.

The occurrence of hemorrhage in thrombocytopenic patients has been shown to be related to the circulating platelet count (GAYDOS *et al.*, 1962). We have demonstrated in this study that platelets obtained from HL-A compatible unrelated donors will effectively increase the platelet count. It may therefore be expected that severe bleeding complications can be reduced in alloimmunized patients with platelet transfusions from HL-A compatible donors. This is further suggested by the fact that none of our 15 patients died of hemorrhage. The patients reported previously (YANKEE *et al.*, 1973) and in this communication have been supported effectively (i. e. without clinically significant bleeding), for up to 9 months with platelets from the same HL-A compatible donor(s). Platelet support with HL-A compatible donors may be especially valuable and rewarding in patients with marrow aplasia or with inactive hematological malignancy (such as "smouldering" leukemia and preleukemia), since the prognosis of these diseases is mainly determined by the quality and efficiency of the transfusion support.

References

ADNER, M. M., FISCH, G. R., STAROBIN, S. G., ASTER, R. H.: Use of "compatible" platelet transfusions in treatment of congenital isoimmune thrombocytopenic purpura. New Engl. J. Med. **280,** 244 (1969).

ALVARADO, J., DJERASSI, I., FARBER, S.: Transfusion of fresh concentrated platelets to children with acute leukemia. J. Pediat. **67,** 13 (1965).

ASTER, R. H.: Effect of anticoagulant and ABO incompatibility on recovery of transfused human platelets. Blood **26,** 732 (1965).

BALDINI, M., COSTEA, N., EBBE, S.: Studies on the antigenic structure of blood platelets, p. 378. 8th Congr. Europ. Soc. Hemat., Vienna, 1961. Basel: Karger 1962.

BRECHER, G., CRONKITE, E. P.: Morphology and enumeration of human blood platelets. J. appl. Physiol. **3,** 365 (1950).

CAVINS, J. A., FARBER, S., ROY, A. J.: Transfusion of fresh platelet concentrates to adult patients with thrombocytopenia. Transfusion **8,** 24 (1968).

CHAPPELL, W. S.: Platelet concentrates from acidified plasma: A method of preparation without the use of additives. Transfusion **6,** 308 (1966).

DAUSSET, J., TANGUN, Y.: Leucocyte and platelet groups and their practical significance. Vox Sang (Basel) **10,** 641 (1965).

DAUSSET, J., COLOMBANI, J., LEGRAND, L., FELLOUS, M.: Genetics of the HL-A system. Deduction of 480 haplotypes. Histocompatibility Testing 1970, p. 53—75. Copenhagen: Munksgaard 1970.

DJERASSI, I., FARBER, S., EVANS, A. E.: Transfusions of fresh platelet concentrates to patients with secondary thrombocytopenia. New Engl. J. Med. **268,** 221 (1963).

FREIREICH, E. J.: Effectiveness of platelet transfusion in leukemia and aplastic anemia. Transfusion **6,** 50 (1966).

FREIREICH, E. J., KLIMAN, A., GAYDOS, L. A., MANTEL, N., FREI, E. III: Response to repeated platelet transfusion from the same donor. Ann. intern. Med. **59,** 277 (1963).

GAYDOS, L. A., FREIREICH, E. J., MANTEL, N.: The quantitative relation between platelet count and hemorrhage in patients with acute leukemia. New Engl. J. Med. **266,** 905 (1962).

GRUMET, F. C., YANKEE, R. A.: Long-term platelet support of patients with aplastic anemia. Effect of splenectomy and steroid therapy. Ann. intern. Med. **73,** 1 (1970).

HAN, T., STUTZMAN, L., COHEN, E., KIM, U.: Effect of platelet transfusion on hemorrhage in patients with acute leukemia. An autopsy study. Cancer **19,** 1937 (1966).

MITTAL, K. K., MICKEY, M. R., SENGAL, D. P., TERASAKI, P. I.: Serotyping for homotransplantation. XVIII. Refinement of microdroplet lymphocyte cytotoxicity test. Transplantation **6,** 913 (1968).

PFISTERER, H., THIERFELDER, S., THIEDE, C., STICH, W.: ABO blood groups and platelet transfusions. Blut **17,** 1 (1968).

Sendroy, J., Jr., Cecchini, L. P.: Determination of human body surface area from height and weight. J. appl. Physiol. **7**, 1 (1954).

Shulman, N. R.: Immunological considerations attending platelet transfusion. Transfusion **6**, 39 (1966).

Shulman, N. R., Marder, V. J., Hiller, M. C., Collier, E. M.: Platelet and leukocyte isoantigens and their antibodies: serologic, physiologic and clinical studies. Progr. Hemat. **4**, 222 (1964).

Svejgaard, A.: Iso-antigenic systems of human blood platelets. A survey. Series Hematol. **II/3**, 29 (1969).

Thorsby, E., Helgesen, A., Gjemdal, T.: Repeated platelet transfusions from HL-A compatible unrelated and sibling donors. Tissue Antigens **2**, 397 (1972).

Yankee, R. A., Grumet, F. C., Rogentine, G. N.: Platelet transfusion therapy. The selection of compatible platelet donors for refractory patients by lymphocyte HL-A typing. New Engl. J. Med. **281**, 1208 (1969).

Yankee, R. A., Leventhal, B. G., Halterman, R. H.: Response to single donor platelet transfusions and *in vitro* tests of alloimmunization. Abstract presented at the Amer. Soc. Hemat. San Francisco, Calif.: Dec. 1971.

Yankee, R. A., Graff, K. S., Dowling, R., Henderson, E. S.: The selection of unrelated compatible platelet donors by lymphocyte HL-A matching. New Engl. J. Med. **288**, 760 (1973).

Immune Responsiveness in Acute Lymphocytic Leukemia Patients under Chemotherapy and Immunotherapy: A Preliminary Report

J. Breard, R. S. Weiner [1], R. K. Oldham [2], and G. Mathé

Institut de Cancérologie et d'Immunogénétique, Hôpital Paul-Brousse, Villejuif

Introduction

With increased survival and prolonged chemotherapy of acute lymphocytic leukemia there have arisen new complications of infection by viral fungal and protozoan organisms which have resulted in significant morbidity and mortality, probably directly related to the immunosuppressive effects of tumoricidal therapy. In assessing new drug regimens for ALL their propensity to cause immunosuppression and the consequences thereof must be evaluated along with the classical parameters of hematologic and organ toxicity and therapeutic effectiveness. We have established and rendered operational a multiphasic schema of immunological evaluation comprising both *in vitro* and *in vivo* tests of cellular immune responsiveness. We report here our early results of the immunologic evaluation of patients during 2 phases of a new protocol for the treatment of acute lymphocytic leukemia, ICIG # 9. For comparison, we report as well the preliminary results of the same battery of tests applied to a group of patients currently under treatment with immunostimulatory therapy for periods of 1—7 years.

Materials and Methods

Patient selection: all patients with newly diagnosed acute lymphocytic leukemia treated at the Institut de Cancérologie et d'Immunogénétique and begun on protocol from November 1, 1972 to April 30, 1973, were eligible. All patients were skin tested and *in vitro* studies were done on those patients whose hematologic status permitted phlebotomy. Patients were tested 6 weeks after complete hematologic remission was obtained and again 12 days after chemotherapy was stopped prior to the initiation of immunotherapy. The interval between the 2 testing periods was 6 months. A final group, who had stopped receiving chemotherapy and had begun immuno-

---

[1] Present Address: Children's Cancer Research Foundation, Boston, MA.
[2] Present Address: National Cancer Institute, Laboratory of Cell Biology. Bethesda, MD.

therapy from 1—7 years prior to testing, was studied once during their course of immunostimulation. The time of testing relative to drug therapy is presented in Table 1.

Table 1. Phases of immunologic evaluation relative to length of complete remission and concurrent therapy

	Time from induction of complete remission	Therapy
Phase 1	4—6 weeks	6 mercaptopurine 50 mg/m²/d p. o. Methotrexate 15 mg/m² i.m. twice weekly Methotrexate 5—10 mg intrathecally
Phase 2	30—32 weeks	12 days after the last of 8—12 cycles of the following: Vincristine 1 mg/m² i.v. days (1 and 2) Methotrexate 20 mg/m² i.v. or i.m. q 6 h for 48 hrs (days 3—4)
Phase 3	2—8 years	BCG (Institut Pasteur) 150 mg by scarification weekly 4×10^7 inactivated pooled allogeneic leukemic blasts subcutaneously — monthly

In vivo tests: The following intradermal skin tests were applied in 0.1 ml and 0.05 ml quantities: Tuberculin (Institut Pasteur) 10 units per 0.1 ml; candidine (Institut Pasteur) 1 to 10,000 dilution; mumps (Ely Lilly) standard dose. Alternate patients were sensitized to DNFB (Merck) either during Phase 1 or Phase 2 of the immunologic testing by topical application in a 2 cm diameter ring. Two thousand micrograms was the sensitizing dose; 100 micrograms was the testing dose applied 14 days later. Picryl chloride was used rather than DNFB on patients undergoing long-term immunostimulation.

In vitro tests: Peripheral blood was drawn into syringes containing preservative-free heparin (Weddel Pharmaceuticals) in a final concentration of 20 units/ml of peripheral blood. The blood was then diluted with 3 volumes of PBS. 35 milliliters of the diluted blood was layered over 15 ml of 8% Ficol (Sigma), 36% Sodium metrizoate (Nyegaard, and Co., Oslo, Norway), specific gravity 1.078 and the lymphocytes separated according to the method of Boyum (1968) in a 50 ml conical centrifuge tube (Falcon 2070). After washing, the cell button was resuspended in 2 ml of media 199 supplemented with glutamine, 4 mg % gentamycin, 25 mmol hepes and 20% homologous decomplemented fresh AB serum. Cell counts were done in a chamber and cell viability determined by the exclusion of trypan blue; cell concentrations were adjusted to 10^6 live lymphocytes per ml.

Concentrations of mitogens: PHA (Difco purified PHA) was used in concentrations of 3 μl/ml.

Pokeweed mitogen (Gibco) was used in concentrations of 62.5 μg/ml.

Microculture: 10^5 lymphocytes in 0.1 ml of complete media were pipetted into each well of a Micro Test II Tissue Culture Plate (Falcon, 3040) and 0.05 ml of the appropriate solution of mitogen added to the wells. The plates were covered with a loose fitting plastic lid (Falcon 3041) wrapped in Saran Wrap and incubated at 37 °C for 72 hrs in a well humidified atmosphere of air.

Thymidine pulsing: Tritiated thymidine (Centre d'Energie Atomique, France) was added to all cultures (0.2 μCi of tritiated thymidine in a volume of 0.05 ml) 6 hrs prior to the end of their incubation.

Extraction: At the end of the incubation period, the cultures were extracted using the MASH I extractor (Microbiological Associates). This machine aspirates the contents of each well and deposits it on a Reeve-Angel fiberglass strip. The apparatus then rinses each well with normal saline and aspirates the rinse, washing the filter paper. After drying to remove water, the filter paper disks were punched out and placed in polyethylene counting vials. 10 ml of scintillation cocktail (PPO 0.5%, POPOP 0.05% in scintillation grade toluene) were added. After equilibration in a dark, cold environment, the samples were counted in a Packard 3375 scintillation spectrometer. All cultures were done in triplicate. Triplicate counts varied maximally 15% above and below the mean value.

Results

Criteria for evaluation of response: Intradermal skin tests were evaluated as positive if induration measured greater than 5 mm. DNFB was positive either spontaneously; *i. e.*, induration or vesiculation arising 9—14 days after the application of the sensitizing dose, or positive on challenge, *i. e.*, induration or vesiculation arising 48—96 hrs after the challenge dose in the absence of spontaneous positivity. Picryl chloride positivity was evaluated by the same criteria. *In vitro* response was evaluated as normal if the mean CPM fell within 50% of the mean CPM of the normal controls cultured on the same day or low if the mean CPM was less than 50% of the mean CPM of the concurrently cultured controls.

In vivo tests: Table 2 shows the results of *in vivo* testing of the three groups of patients. We have defined anergy as the absence of a delayed hypersensitivity response to any of the three recall antigens and primary sensitization antigen applied to the patient. The most striking results are the high incidence of anergy in those patients under continuous combination chemotherapy and the absence of anergy in those evaluated within the 3 weeks following the last course of intermittent chemotherapy and during the prolonged immunostimulatory period. The successful primary sensitization to DNFB in 2 patients in the group under continuous chemotherapy emphasizes the heterogeneity of reactivity within the group. The 25% incidence of response to picryl chloride sensitization in the immunotherapy group may indicate a hyper-reactivity within that group since the response to picryl chloride in other groups of untreated cancer patients is negative or negligible (BLUMING *et al.*, 1972).

In vitro tests: Table 3 shows our results of *in vitro* correlates of immune reactivity by mitogen stimulation. There is a steady increase in the incidence of normal responsiveness from the continuous chemotherapy to the end of intermittent chemotherapy through immunotherapy in the groups tested. The differences are not statistically significant, however. Further, we have shown recently (WEINER *et al.*, 1973)

Table 2. Delayed cutaneous hypersensitivity. Patients were skin tested with antigens during continuous maintenance chemotherapy (Phase 1); 12 days after the last course of intermittent chemotherapy (Phase 2); and during immunostimulatory therapy of 1—7 years duration (Phase 3). Responses to tuberculin, Candida, and mumps were scored as positive if induration was 5 mm or more in diameter. Responses to DNFB and Picryl Chloride were scored as positive if induration and/or vesiculation occurred either 9—14 days after primary sensitization or 72—96 hours after challenge

	N° Positive / N° Tested					N° Anergic [b] / Total
	Tuberculin	Candida	Mumps	DNFB [a]	Picryl Chloride	
Phase 1	5/21	4/21	2/21	2/11		14/21
Phase 2	7/15	7/15	2/15	1/10		0/15
Phase 3	23/23	9/23	9/23		6/23	0/23

[a] Randomized DNFB or non-DNFB at Phase 1. Non-DNFB given DNFB at Phase 2.
[b] No positive skin tests.

Table 3. *In vitro* lymphocyte stimulation. Patients lymphocytes were stimulated with PHA and with PWM during continuous maintenance chemotherapy (Phase 1); 12 days after the last course of intermittent maintenance chemotherapy (Phase 2); and during immunostimulatory therapy of 1—7 years duration (Phase 3). Responses were scored as "normal" if the mean incorporation of thymidine as counts per minute were within 50% of the mean values of "normal" lymphocytes tested on the same day. Those values less than 50% of the normal were scored as "low"

		N° Responding / N° Tested		
		Phase 1	Phase 2	Phase 3
PHA	Normal	4/8	8/11	13/17
	Low	4/8	3/11	4/17
PWM	Normal	3/8	6/11	12/17
	Low	5/8	5/11	5/17

valid longitudinal comparisons are difficult with *in vitro* tests because of the day-to-day variability in response. We chose as a standard, the reactivity of the normal lymphocytes cultured on the same day, but we acknowledge that the limits we set for the normal reactivity are arbitrary. Our current studies involve cryopreserved lymphocytes, allowing us to evaluate changes in the patients' lymphocyte reactivity with time and therapy.

Discussion

It is widely accepted that intermittent chemotherapy is less immunosuppressive than continuous chemotherapy. That immunostimulatory therapy may increase the responsiveness to a weak antigen was reported by Bluming *et al.* (1972), and our data confirm their observations with respect to picryl chloride as well. The battery of skin tests used to assess delayed cutaneous hypersensitivity is valid in France, especially since BCG immunization is supposedly universal by school age. The patients studied were within that age group with two exceptions. The *in vitro* results reported included only mitogen stimulation since those were the tests which were technically reliable at the time of the study. We have since expanded the *in vitro* battery to include stimulation by PPD and by defined populations of allogeneic cells. The *in vitro* assessment of cellular immune responsiveness is a subject of active research and any protocol designed to evaluate changes in cellular immunity must evolve as new information becomes available. The use of cryopreserved lymphocytes will aid in defining changes in the individual patient. The ability to separate the subpopulations of immunoresponsive cells eventually will permit more precise definition of the effects of disease and therapy on host responses.

The preliminary studies reported herein illustrate the feasibility of studying the effects of therapy on immunologic responsiveness. Such routine evaluation in as detailed a manner as possible should be included in the experimental design of all new protocols subjected to Phase II or Phase III trials.

References

Bluming, A. Z., Vogel, C. L., Ziegler, J. L., Mody, N., Kamya, G.: Immunologic effects of BCG therapy in malignant melanoma: Two modes of therapy compared. Ann. intern. Med. **76**, 405 (1972).

Boyum, A.: Separation of leukocytes from blood and bone marrow. Scand. J. clin. Lab. Invest. **21**, 77 (1968).

Weiner, R. S., Breard, J., O'Brien, C.: Use of cryopreserved lymphocytes in sequential studies of immunoresponsiveness, p. 117. In: CRYOPRESERVATION OF NORMAL AND NEOPLASTIC CELLS. Ed.: R. S. Weiner, R. K. Oldham, L. Schwartzenberg. Paris: I.N.S.E.R.M. 1973.

Abbreviations

BCG — Bacillus Calmette-Guerin
PHA — Phytohemagglutinin
PWM — Pokeweed mitogen
ALL — Acute lymphocytic leukemia
DNFB — Dinitrofluorobenzene
CPM — Counts per minute
PBS — Phosphate buffered saline

Transfer Factor Therapy in Immunodeficiencies*

C. GRISCELLI [1], H. BETUEL [2], C. HERZOG [1], J. L. TOURAINE [3], and J. P. REVILLARD [3]

Unité d'Hématologie et Immunologie Infantiles, Clinique Médicale Infantile, INSERM U 132 Hôpital Necker-Enfants Malades, Paris [1], Centre de Transfusion Sanguine de Lyon, Beynost [2], and Clinique de Néphrologie et des Maladies Métaboliques et groupe I.N.S.E.R.M. U 80, Hôpital de l'Anticaille, Lyon [3]

Abstract

Dialysable Transfer Factor was prepared from a large pool of normal adult donor leukocytes following Lawrence's technique. This homogeneous preparation was injected into 3 normal recipients and 14 patients with immunodeficiencies: 5 ataxia telangiectasia, 4 Wiskott-Aldrich syndrome, 2 variable hypogammaglobulinemia, 2 combined immunodeficiencies and one chronic mucocutaneous candidiasis. Transfer of delayed hypersensitivity of several antigenic markers was achieved in 13 cases. Streptokinase — streptodornase and *Candida albicans* gave the highest incidence of positive tests among adult donors and recipients. 5 recipients developed a positive reaction to DNCB, a chemical to which none of the donors was sensitized.

Clinical improvement was observed in only 2 cases of Wiskott-Aldrich syndrome. Therapeutic effects were absent or uncertain in the other cases.

Antigen-induced lymphocyte proliferation *in vitro* was modified in only 4 cases. If confirmed, the apparent dissociations between skin reactions, blast transformation and clinical improvement in recipients of transfer factor would suggest that transfer factor may also act by inducing the peripheral manifestation of a cellular hypersensitivity already acquired although not expressed by the immunologically deficient recipient.

The successful transfer of cell-mediated hypersensitivity to tuberculin and streptococcal antigens in man was first achieved by LAWRENCE (1949). In contrast to similar experiments in the guinea pig (CHASE, 1945), cellular transfer in humans requires a relatively small number of leukocytes. Moreover, the duration of the transferred sensitivity was usually much greater than the survival of intact leukocytes in a histo-incompatible host. This observation suggested that the active principle might survive the immunological rejection of the transferred cells. In several experiments designed to characterize the active material, LAWRENCE showed that effective transfer

* Supported in part by Foundation pour la Recherche Médicale et Scientifique, Paris, and INSERM.

of delayed-type hypersensitivity could be achieved with disrupted leukocytes and even with the dialysable moiety of frozen and thawed DNAase-treated leukocytes. This dialysable active material was called "transfer factor" by LAWRENCE. It is soluble, lyophilizable, and heat-sensitive; it resists pancreatic RNAase, and retains its potency after 5 years of storage; its estimated molecular weight is below 10,000 (LAWRENCE, 1960).

Defects in delayed cutaneous hypersensitivity in a variety of diseases can be associated with defects in "cellular immunity" that lead to repeated severe infections by fungi or intracellular parasites, such as viruses and some bacteria (MACKANESS, 1967; MAUPIN, 1959; PABST and SWANSON, 1972; PREUD'HOMME *et al.*, in press; ROCKLIN *et al.*, 1970; SCHULKIND *et al.*, 1972; SØBORG *et al.*, 1971; SPITLER *et al.*, 1971, 1972 a+b; TOURAINE and REVILLARD, 1970 and in press; VALDIMARSSON *et al.*, 1972; VALENTINE and LAWRENCE, 1971). Attempts to transfer delayed hypersensitivity by means of intact leukocytes or dialysable transfer factor have been successful in most patients, and a classification of cellular defects according to the result

Table 1. Wiskott-Aldrich Syndrome: Clinical and biological data in 4 TF recipients

Patients	WA 1	WA 2	WA 3	WA 4
Age	9	$5^1/_2$	11	4
Hemorrhages	++	++	++	++
Eczema	mild	chronic	none	mild
Infections	+++	+++	++	++
Arthralgia	+	+	0	0
Splenomegaly	0	+	0	0
Platelets $10^3/mm^3$	50	20—50	10—40	20—40
Cellular defect	++	++	+	±
IgM mg/ml	0.14	0.45	0.1	0.5
IgA mg/ml	2.85	4.27	1.65	2.3
TF injections (units)	1 × 3	1 × 3	1	1
Clinical improvement	yes	yes	no	no

of the transfer has been proposed (for review see LAWRENCE, 1969). In Hodgkin's disease, for example, the transfer of local or systemic hypersensitivity nearly always failed, whereas in sarcoidosis the transfer of local sensitivity could be achieved, although systemic sensitivity was not usually demonstrable. Generalized vaccinia was cured upon transfer of viable leukocytes from a hypersensitive donor where repeated injections of hyperimmune globulins had been ineffective (LAWRENCE, 1969 a). Delayed hypersensitivity to *Candida albicans* was acquired in patients with chronic mucocutaneous candidiasis following transfer of a parental bone marrow graft (BUCKLEY, 1968) or after injections of dialysable transfer factor prepared from hypersensitive donors (McFARLIN and OPPENHEIM, 1969; KIRCKPATRICK *et al.*, 1972; PABST and SWANSON, 1972; ROCKLIN *et al.*, 1970; SCHULKIND *et al.*, 1972). Similarly, the transfer of hypersensitivity to lepromin (antigens to the lepra bacillus) was demonstrated in anergic lepromatous patients receiving leukocytes from sensitive donors (DE BONAPARTE *et al.*, 1968). It is still too early to assess the effects of such successful transfers on the disease itself. However, it was recently shown that the injection of dialysable transfer factor in patients with a Wiskott-Aldrich syndrome resulted both in the conversion of the patient to a hypersensitive state and in an improvement of such clinical manifestations as infections, splenomelagy, hemorrhages and eczema (LEVIN *et al.*, 1970). It has been claimed that the outcome of attempts to treat the Wiskott-Aldrich syndrome with transfer factor can be predicted from a study of the immunoglobulin receptors on the patient's monocytes (SPITLER *et al.*, 1972 a).

In our study, the potential therapeutic value of dialysable transfer factor in various immunodeficiencies of children is evaluated. Dialysable transfer factor was selected because its low molecular weight allows repeated injections into the same recipient without risk of inoculation of viruses or of sensitization to transplantation antigens. To obtain comparable results, this material was prepared from a large pool of normal adult donor leukocytes. Thus, the effectiveness of the transfer will depend on the immune state of the recipient and not on differences between batches of transfer factor.

I. Material and Methods

1. Donors

Healthy adult blood donors free of Australia antigen, were submitted to medical examination. They were skin-tested with the following antigens: tuberculin PPD 0.1 µg (Mérieux), streptokinase-streptodornase (SK-SD, Varidase, Lederle, 10 units), candidin (Institut Pasteur, Paris, 1/10,000), toxoplasmin (1/100); diphtheria toxoid (Mérieux, dose equivalent to 0.6 Lf) and autoclaved vaccinia virus (1/10 of the immunizing dose). Erythema (E) and induration (I) measured at 24 h and 48 h; the intensity of the reaction depends mainly on the dose of antigen injected. In this series we found 52% of donors positive to PPD, 48% to candidin, 85% to SK-SD, 90% to vaccinia, 18% to toxoplasmin and 25% to diphtheria toxoid. The donors were not tested with DNCB, since none of them had a history of sensitization to this chemical.

2. Preparation of Transfer Factor (TF)

Ten blood units are collected on citric acid-citrate-dextrose, centrifuged for 30 min at 1000 g, the plasma layer is discarded and the buffy coat treated according to Maupin's technique of "paradoxical" sedimentation (MAUPIN, 1959). The buffy coat is spun at 500 g, then a 50% glucose solution is introduced through the bottom of the flask; this allows the recovery of four layers: (1) plasma, (2) platelets, (3) white blood cells, (4) red cells and a few leukocytes. The third layer is washed with saline and centrifuged at 300 g for 3 min. White cells are counted and the cell pellet is then frozen and thawed (10 cycles), DNase (1 mg to 4 ml packed cells) being added at the second cycle. This material is dialyzed for 3 days against distilled water through a double cuprophane membrane (Travenol UF 100). The dialysate is lyophilized, then pooled and redissolved in distilled water to lower the osmolarity to a maximum of 650 mOsm, passed through two millipore filters (0.45 µm and 0.30 µm). One unit is defined as the final product of 6×10^9 leukocytes, its average volume is 5 ml. The following checks are made on each batch before clinical use: bacteriological evaluation (15 days at 4 °C, 20 °C and 37 °C) including cultures on Sabouraud's medium; absence of soluble HL-A antigens as shown by absorption methods on monospecific HL-A antisera; absence of toxic effects on guinea pigs after injection of 0.2 ml s.c. on donors (see Table 3) and also with 0.5% DNCB (Lawrence, 1963), *Aspergillus fumigatus* and *Aspergillus nidulans*. Proliferative responses of blood lymphocytes to mitogens (PHA P, Difco 1/200—1/800, ALS) and dialysed antigens (PPD 1 μg/ml, Candidin 1/1200—1/2800, SK-SD 200 U/ml) were assessed by measuring the incorporation of ^{3}H-thymidine into DNA according to a technique previously described (Brochier, 1971). Cultures were performed in 20% heat-inactivated AB serum and results were expressed in dpm/10^6 lymphocytes. A leukocyte migration test was performed according to Søborg's method (1971). The following antigens were used at different concentrations: PPD, SK-SD and streptococcal wall.

3. Recipients

1—3 units of TF were injected into 3 normal subjects and 14 patients with immunodeficiency classified according to WHO recommendations.

a) *Three normal subjects* were examined and subjected to routine laboratory investigation; this showed no evidence of patent or latent disease.

NS 1 is a healthy 24-year-old female who exhibited no skin reaction to 5 μg PPD after 4 subsequent tests, despite a BCG vaccination at the age of 9.

NS 2 is a 10-year-old boy who had no BCG vaccination and negative skin reaction to 5 μg PPD.

NS 3 is a 7-year-old girl with skin tests repeatedly negative to PPD (5 μg) and SK-SD (100 U) but positive for candidin.

b) *Wiskott-Aldrich syndrome* (W.A.). 4 boys presenting the typical clinical and biological manifestations of W.A. syndrome are recorded in Table 1. Nasopharyngeal and cutaneous infections were predominant. Cellular defect was considered more or less pronounced according to skin tests and proliferative responses to mitogens "*in vitro*".

c) *Ataxia Telangiectasia* (AT) (Table 2). 5 children suffering from AT received TF injections. All these patients showed ocular telangiectasia; all had presented with

Table 2. Ataxia Telangiectasia: Clinical and biological data in 5 patients

Patient	AT 1	AT 2	AT 3	AT 4	AT 5
Sex	F.	M.	F.	M.	F.
Age	$3^1/_2$	$4^1/_2$	7	9	4
Ataxia	+	+	+	+	+
Polyneuritis	+	+	0	0	0
Infections	++	++	++	+++	+++
Cellular defect	++	++	±	++	++
IgA mg/ml	< 0.1	0.6	< 0.1	< 0.1	< 0.1
Injections (units)	1 × 3	1 × 3	1 × 3	1	1
Clinical improvement	partial	partial	partial	no	no

repeated episodes of nasopharyngeal and bronchial infections which had resulted in diffuse bronchiectasis. No gastrointestinal infections were recorded. A plasma factor inhibiting lymphocyte responses to mitogens was detected in 3 cases (AT 1, AT 2, AT 3), as previously reported by MacFarlin *et al.*, 1969.

d) *Combined immunodeficiency* (CID) *CID 1.* This 6-month-old girl, whose brother and sister died of infection under one year of age, presented severe lymphopenia (180/mm^3) and a marked cellular defect with no response to mitogens *in vitro.* Immunoglobulin levels were: IgG 2.8 mg/ml, IgA 0.6 mg/ml, IgM 0.88 mg/ml. No antibody response was obtained after various attempts at stimulation. She received 2 doses of TF 2 months apart.

CID 2. This 8-month-old boy had 2 meningitic infections caused by *Listeria monocytogenes* at 5 and 6 months. He presented a moderate lymphopenia (1200/mm^3) and a profound cellular defect with no *in vitro* response to mitogens (PHA and ALS). Immunoglobulin levels were: IgG 2.4 mg/ml, IgA 0.10 mg/ml, IgM 0.23 mg/ml; no antibody response was obtained. He received a single dose of TF. Among uncles and great uncles on the maternal side there were 10 early deaths due to infections.

e) *Variable hypogammaglobulinemia* (VH). Two hypogammaglobulinemia patients with no family record of immunodeficiency were treated:

VH 1. A 10-year-old boy, had severe, repeated pulmonary infections and meningitis starting at the age of 3 months. He had measles at 5$^1/_2$ years. Later he developed progressive encephalitis. Evidence of leukoencephalitis was apparent on a brain biopsy specimen, and tubular granules were observed in the cytoplasm of endothelial cells of cerebral capillaries by electron microscopy (Lyon *et al.*, 1972). Immunoglobulin levels were very low: IgG 2.9 mg/ml, IgA 0.1 mg/ml, IgM 0.05 mg/ml. Membrane immunoglobulins were detected on peripheral blood lymphocytes; however, only 3% stained for IgG, 0.02% for IgM and 0.01% for IgA (Preud'homme *et al.*, in press). No significant antibody response was observed following vaccinations. Although suspected from the clinical data, no cellular immunological defect was ascertained. This patient received two consecutive injections of TF 4 months apart.

VH 2. A 14-year-old boy, had suffered from repeated cutaneous, bronchial and nasopharyngeal infections since early infancy. He had no detectable cellular defect and had recovered normally from viral infections. Serum immunoglobulin levels were very low: IgG 3.0 mg/ml, IgA 0.1 mg/ml, IgM 0.08 mg/ml. Almost no blood lymphocytes bearing membrane immunoglobulins could be seen. This patient received two injections of TF 3 months apart.

f) *Chronic mucocutaneous candidiasis* (CC). This 16-year-old girl had severe chronic mucocutaneous candidiasis and bronchiectasis (Touraine and Revillard, 1970). There was no family history of candidiasis or immunodeficiency, no abnormality of adrenal or parathyroid functions. Serum immunoglobulin concentrations were normal and anti-candidin antibodies were present. She had relapsed after two treatments with amphotericin B and her skin tests had been repeatedly negative to candidin. PHA response *in vitro* was normal. She received 5 doses of TF over 5 months. No anti-moniliasis therapy was given during this period.

II. Results

1. Clinical Tolerance

The site of TF injection was painful for 30 min; after that no local or systemic reaction was observed, even upon repeated injections. Of interest was the absence of fever in 16 recipients. A slight rise in lymphocyte and monocyte counts was recorded in an occasional recipient (WA 1, WA 2, AT 1, AT 2, VH 1, VH 2). No late side-effect was reported on 12-month follow-up. In one patient (WA 2) fever, arthralgia, and enlargement of spleen and lymph nodes were observed transiently 8 days after TF injection and 24 h after infusion of cesium-irradiated histoincompatible blood. This patient had received multiple transfusions. No adverse reaction was observed after two other TF injections.

2. Delayed Hypersensitivity

No significant change was seen in skin reactions in NS 2, VH 2, CID 1 and 2, and AT 5. In the 12 other recipients changes in delayed skin reactions were observed (Table 3). The most significant modifications occurred with SK-SD and candidin. Local transfer was successful in 9 instances (7 patients). Systemic transfer was less easily achieved; a positive response was elicited with only one or two of the 8 antigens under investigation and was usually of short duration, except with NS 1 and CC who received 5 injections of TF.

Contact sensitivity to DNCB (Table 4) became positive in 5 recipients (WA 1, WA 2, AT 1, AT 3, AT 5). All had been sensitized to DNCB (15% in acetone) and had shown at least two negative reactions to the test dose (0.5% in acetone). Although no skin biopsy was performed, the positive reactions observed after injection of TF showed the typical aspect of a delayed reaction. In 3 cases (WA 4, AT 2, VH 1) a stronger reaction to 0.5% DNCB was observed after injection of TF.

3. Leukocyte Migration and Lymphocyte Transformation

In 8 patients, leukocyte migration tests were performed on 2—4 blood samples taken at different times before injection of TF. Because of considerable spontaneous variation in the concentrations of antigens inhibiting the migration, the effect of TF injection could not be evaluated with this test.

No significant change of the PHA response *in vitro* was recorded after injection of TF in 3 normal subjects and 11 patients. However, the 3 patients with a PHA response either very low (AT 4) or absent (WA 2, AT 1) showed a significant rise in proliferative response to this mitogen 8 days after injection of TF (Table 5). It was transient in patient AT and longer-lasting in patients WA 2 and AT 1. Normal laboratory values are between 50,000 and 150,000 dpm/10^6 cells.

Modifications of antigen-induced lymphocyte proliferation were observed in a few cases (Table 6). In normal subjects with positive skin tests, the *in vitro* response was increased in NS 1 (SK-SD), NS 2 (cand., SK-SD) and NS 3 (cand.), even when the size of the skin reaction was unchanged (NS 2). Lymphocytes from NS 3 did

Table 3. Changes in skin reactions after injection of TF[a]

Patient	Antigen	Dose	Before	24 h local	24 h systemic	Day 8	Day 23—50	Day 80—180
NS 1	PPD	5 µG	0 < 0	10— 8	12—10	20—10	10— 8	5— 4
NS 3	CAND	1/100	12—16	ND	53—36	ND	ND	ND
	SK-SD	10 u	0 0	ND	21— 7	17—11	7— 5	ND
WA 1	CAND	1/1000	0 0	ND	0 0	7— 6	8— 7	0— 0
	SK-SD	20	0 0	ND	0 0	13—11	8— 7	0— 0
WA 2	CAND	1/1000	0 0	ND	0 0	0 0	6— 4	0 0
	PPD	1 µG	0 0	9— 9	0 0	0 0	0 0	0 0
WA 3	CAND	1/1000	0 0	ND	0 0	33—12	ND	0 0
	PPD	1 µG	0 0	6— 4	0 0	0 0	ND	0 0
	SK-SD	20	0 0	6— 6	0 0	0 0	ND	0 0
WA 4	ASP N	0.1	0 0	ND	0 0	0 0	20—18	ND
	ASP F	0.1	0 0	ND	0 0	0 0	11—10	ND
AT 1	CAND	1/1000	4— 0	ND	13— 9	0 0	0 0	ND
AT 2	CAND	1/1000	0 0	6— 5	0 0	0 0	0 0	0 0
AT 3	SK-SD	20	0 0	7— 5	12— 0	12— 5	30—15	ND
	CAND	1/1000	0 0	9— 5	0 0	0 0	5— 0	ND
AT 4	SK-SD	20	0 0	6— 4	5— 0	10— 0	0 0	ND
VH 1	DIPH TOX	0.6	0 0	ND	12— 6	0 0	0 0	ND
CC	CAND	1/100	5— 5	ND	52—21	36—16	32—14	44—22
	CAND	1/1000	4— 4	20—10	20—10	10— 7	11— 5	26—11
	SK-SD	10	5— 0	ND	12— 3	30—12	9— 4	12— 7
	VACCINIA	1/10	2— 4	ND	17— 4	11— 6	9— 7	4— 4

[a] In each column the mean diameters of erythema (left) and induration (right) are measured in mm. ND: not done.

Table 4. Contact sensitivity to DNCB (0.5%) in recipients of TF[a]

Patient	Before	24 h	Day 8	Day 23—50	Day 80—180
WA 1	0— 0	0— 0	0— 0	11—10	0— 0
WA 2	0— 0	5— 5	6— 5	13—10	0— 0
AT 1	0— 0	5— 5	7— 6	20—20	20—15
AT 3	0— 0	6— 0	6— 0	10— 5	ND
AT 5	0— 0	6— 0	6— 0	11— 6	ND
WA 4	7—11	11— 9	ND	20—12	ND
AT 2	9— 7	30—15	22—22	22—22	ND
VH 1	5— 5	ND	9— 6	40—30	ND

[a] In each column the mean diameters of erythema (left) and induration (right) are measured in mm. ND: not done.

Table 5. Changes in the PHA response in recipients of TF. Results in dpm/10^6 lymphocytes

Patient	Stimulant	Before	Day 8	Day 30—80
WA 2	PHA 1/600	1100	15649	18794
	0	920	1459	1271
AT 1	PHA 1/600	1000	6400	13000
	0	816	1400	1341
AT 4	PHA 1/600	3700	13896	4504
	0	1286	493	1430

Table 6. Incorporation of ^{3}H-thymidine in dpm/tube measured at day 6 before and after injection of TF

Patient	Antigen	Dose	Before	Day 3	Day 30—80
NS 1	0		1012	1348	1972
	PPD	5 µg/ml	3473	4641	8559
	SK-SD	400 U/ml	6010	14496	46501
NS 2	0		173	150	504
	CAND	1/1200	820	895	36396
	SK-SD	400 U/ml	531	650	3647
NS 3	0		1055	32	1533
	PPD	5 µg/ml	664	1383	6121
	CAND	1/1200	160	740	35526
	SK-SD	400 µ/ml	1225	2450	11610
WA 4	0		815	1684	802
	SK-SD	500 u/ml	1291	7047	1624
	CAND	1/2000	807	2678	873
AT 3	0		2557	1528	1064
	PPD	10 µg/ml	4710	8056	17049
	SK-SD	100 u/ml	2448	ND	23976
VH 2	0		2022	2010	678
	SK-SD	400 u/ml	15260	47388	8121
	CAND	1/2800	3922	8908	1252
CC	0		2327	2907	2987
	CAND	1/200	2800	10065	10358
	SK-SD	200 u/ml	5929	4856	22124

not respond to candidin before injection of TF, despite a positive skin reaction (Table 3); such a dissociation between *in vivo* and *in vitro* reactions of normal subjects is highly exceptional in our laboratory. Conversion to a hypersensitive state was associated with the development (NS 3 : SK-SD) or the increase (NS 1 : PPD) of a proliferative response to the corresponding antigen. A slight increase in the *in vitro* response to PPD was noticed in NS 3 despite the absence of a demonstrable skin reaction to this antigen. *In vitro* responses to antigenic stimulation remained absent in 9 patients with immunodeficiency (WA 1, WA 2, WA 3, AT 1, AT 2, AT 4, AT 5, VH 1, CID 1 and CID 2); among this group of patients, 6 acquired delayed hypersensitivity to one or several of the antigens tested *in vitro* (Table 3). Patient WA 4 showed a slight increase of his responses to SK-SD and candidin (Table 6) but without a demonstrable skin reaction to these antigens. Patient AT 3, who had a very mild cellular defect, acquired a positive *in vitro* response to SK-SD and PPD. Patient VH 2 showed a transient increase of his *in vitro* responses to SK-SD and candidin; his skin reactions to these antigens were positive before the injection of TF. Patient CC converted to a positive *in vivo* and *in vitro* reaction to candidin, and her response to SK-SD was increased (Table 6). In summary, whereas a delayed hypersensitivity skin reaction was demonstrable after injection of TF in 10 patients with immunodeficiency, antigen-induced lymphocyte proliferation *in vitro* was modified in only 4 cases.

4. Effects on Clinical Manifestations

Patients with severe combined immunodeficiency (CID 1, CID 2) did not show any evidence of clinical improvement upon injection of TF. CID 2 was later given a bone marrow transplantation. No change was observed in patients VH 1 and VH 2. Patient CC showed a transient improvement of her oral lesions, without changes in the fingernails but then returned to her initial state despite the presence of a strongly positive skin reaction to candidin. Some improvement was noticed in patients WA 1 and WA 2: decrease of infections, nasal bleeding, splenomegaly and eczema occurred during the 3 months following the two injections of TF. However, as spontaneous variations in clinical manifestations for the same patient do occur in this syndrome, conclusions should not be drawn prematurely. In the three cases AT 1, AT 2 and AT 3, a decrease in the intensity of bronchitis and pharyngitis was noted for 2—3 months after each TF injections, but there was no significant regression of neurological signs.

III. Discussion

Our experience with transfer-factor therapy confirms some of LEVIN's (1970) observations and presents new observations for discussion. The incidence of positive transfers in normal or sick recipients appears lower than in LAWRENCE's experience (1969). In our series, sensitivity to streptokinase and candidin was often acquired or increased in recipients but hypersensitivity to PPD was less often seen. According to LAWRENCE (1969 b), a higher incidence of positive transfers could be achieved if the selection of donors was made on the basis of exquisite hypersensitivity to low doses of antigen. Chromatography of dialysable transfer factor on Sephadex G 25 showed two peaks but only peak II (mol. wt. $< 10{,}000$) transferred coccidioidin sensitivity (LAWRENCE, 1963). Exclusion of inactive material (peak I) from the dialysate might increase the incidence of positive transfers and certainly deserves further laboratory investigation. In some instances dissociation between skin reactivity and the *in vitro* proliferative response of lymphocytes to antigens was observed. Recipient NS 1 did not exhibit any skin reaction to repeated tests with 5 μg of PPD whereas her lymphocytes showed a small but significant response to PPD *in vitro*. It is of interest that transfer factor in this case resulted both in a transient positive skin reaction and in a slight increase of the *in vitro* response. A similar dissociation was observed after injection of TF in WA_4 (SK-SD, cand.) and AT 3 (PPD). Conversely, in 6 patients no significant increase was seen in the proliferative response to antigens but skin reactions were positive. This lack of correlation between *in vivo* and *in vitro* responses to antigens is exceptional in normal subjects but is known to occur in immunodeficient subjects after injection of TF (EIJSVOOGEL, person. commun.; FALL and ZABRISKIE; MCFARLIN and OPPENHEIM, 1969; KIRKPATRICK *et al.*, 1972; LAWRENCE, 1949, 1960, 1963, 1969 a+b; LAWRENCE and FISHMAN, 1972; LEVIN *et al.;* 1970). Measurements of MIF production by the recipient's lymphocytes by the blood leukocyte migration test did not yield significant results in our series. It appears from the published data that transfer factor induces MIF production (EIJSVOOGEL, person. commun.; LEVIN *et al.*, 1970; ROCKLIN *et al.*, 1970) rather than blast transformation in recipients' lymphocytes.

The effect of TF on clinical manifestations in two cases of Wiskott-Aldrich syndrome confirms the original observation of LEVIN *et al.* (1970); SPITLER *et al.* (1972b), as well as other cases recorded by LAWRENCE (1972). The fact that, after regression of infections, eczema and bleeding, patients WA 1 and WA 2 had a relapse, as evidenced by spleen enlargement and recurrence of infections, may suggest the need for repeated injections of TF in such patients. The clinical improvement observed in these 2 patients and in 3 cases of ataxia telangiectasia may have been due to improved host resistance resulting from the induction of effective cellular immunity to the antigens to which the normal adult donors were resistant. However, two unexpected observations argue against this hypothesis and may provide some information about the still unknown mechanism of action of TF. Manifest clinical improvement in patients WA 2 and AT 2 contrasted with little effect, if any, on skin reactions. Furthermore, 5 recipients developed marked hypersensitivity to DNCB, a chemical to which none of the donors was known to be sensitized (Table 4). We cannot exclude the role of repeated testing in the induction of contact sensitivity after injection of TF.

TF is usually regarded as an informational molecule, nucleotide cofactor, or derepressor which transfers the specific sensitivities of the donors. If confirmed, our observations would suggest that TF may also act by inducing the peripheral manifestation of a cellular hypersensitivity already acquired although not expressed by the immunologically deficient recipient. This hypothesis, in contrast with prevailing concepts, deserves further investigation since Lawrence's observations in normal recipients may not be applicable to immunodeficient patients. The use of a large pool of leukocyte donors may allow the transfer of delayed hypersensitivity (evaluated by skin reactions and/or antigen-induced blastogenesis) to be observed with some, but not all, antigens to which the donors were positive. Different responses to the injection of the same pool of TF among patients presenting with the same clinical syndrome undoubtedly reflect differences in severity of illness, or heterogeneity of the syndrome. Discrepancies between clinical improvement and the absence of transfer of delayed skin reactions seem to show that skin testing is not a good indicator of the clinical effect of TF therapy. Moreover, some recipients acquired positive skin tests without any change in the course of their disease (e.g. patient CC had persistent lesions despite a strong skin reaction to candidin). Additional chemotherapy or antibiotic therapy may be beneficial in such cases (SPITLER *et al.*, 1971; VALDIMARSSON *et al.*, 1972).

Controlled clinical trials of TF may help to classify various immunodeficiencies and provide new data for understanding the relationships between delayed hypersensitivity and cellular immunity. TF should certainly be used before any major treatment such as thymus or bone marrow graft.

TF does not carry the risk of sensitization to transplantation antigens nor the hazards of a graft-versus-host reaction, and after more than one year of follow-up no patient had developed hepatitis. In view of the absence of any adverse reaction in recipients of TF in this series, and since the therapeutic effect of this principle is not yet understood, it seems reasonable to investigate its potential therapeutic value in congenital or acquired deficiencies of cellular immunity, despite the rather low incidence and short duration of the clinical effects we observed.

Note of the authors. We have observed recently (C. GRISCELLI, C. MAWAS and P. MOZZICONACCI) a patient with a partial hypogammaglobulinemia and normal proliferation response *in vitro* with various antigens. In contrast, skin reactions with the same antigens at various concentrations were negative.

MIF, mitogenic and chemotactic factors were normally produced. Despite a normal mixed leucocyte reaction (MLR) with non-identical donor stimulating cells, skin graft from the same donor was not rejected. Cellular mediated lymphotoxicity (CML) using allogenic cells from the same donor was considerably decreased. The patient's serum had no blocking effect in MLR and CML.

After the injection of transfer factor, it was possible to obtain, in this patient with a specific defect of cytotoxic effectors, positive skin reactions and inflammatory lesions in the skin graft.

This observation may indicate the transfer factor operates on the expression of the effector cells implicated in delayed hypersensitivity and in skin graft reaction.

Acknowledgements

We thank Dr. MAUPIN and Miss C. CARBONNE for their help in the preparation of TF, Dr. FREYCON carried our the clinical examination of normal recipients. Pr. LARBRE and Dr. FREYCON were responsible for patient CC, and Dr. GILLY of patient VH 2. We thank the physicians who referred their patients to one of us: Pr. D. ALAGILLE (WA 1), Pr. DELAITRE (VA 2), Pr. ROYER (VH 1), Pr. M. SELIGMANN (WA 3, WA 4), Pr. SALET (AT 1, AT 2), Pr. MALLET (AT 5), Pr. FRÉZAL (CID 2), Pr. SANCHEZ Villarez from Valladolid (CID 1). Dr. J. F. BACH performed leukocyte migration tests.

The blood donors and the staff of the Centre de transfusion sanguine, Lyons, who made this study possible deserve our deep appreciation.

References

DE BONAPARTE, Y., MORGENFELD, M. C., PARADISI, E. R.: Immunology of leprosy. New Engl. J. Med. **279**, 49 (1968).

BROCHIER, J.: Mesure de la transformation et de la prolifération des lymphocytes humains en culture. Path. Biol. **19**, 833 (1971).

BUCKLEY, R. H., LUCAS, Z. J., HATTLER, B. G., JR. *et al.:* Defective cellular immunity associated with chronic mucocutaneous moniliasis and recurrent staphylococcal botryomycosis. Immunological reconstitution by allogeneic bone marrow. Clin. exp. Immunol. **3**, 153 (1968).

CHASE, M. W.: The cellular transfer of cutaneous hypersensitivity to tuberculin. Proc. Soc. exp. Bio. (N.Y.) **59**, 134 (1945).

DUPUY, J. M., and PREUD'HOMME, J. L.: Exploration de l'hypersensibilité retardée par le 2,4-dinitrochlorobenzène (D.N.C.B.) Presse Méd. **76**, 123 (1968).

EIJSVOOGEL, V. P.: Personal communication.

FALK, R. E., ZABRISKIE, J. B.: The capillary technique for measurement of inhibition of leukocyte migration. op. Cit. 301.

MCFARLIN, D. E., OPPENHEIM, J. J.: Impaired lymphocyte transformation in ataxia-telangiectasia in part due to a plasma inhibitory factor. J. Immunol. **103**, 1212 (1969).

KIRKPATRICK, C. H., RICH, R. R., and SMITH, T. K.: Effect of transfer factor on lymphocyte function in Anergic Patients. J. clin. Invest. **51**, 2948 (1972).

LAWRENCE, H. S.: The cellular transfer of cutaneous hypersensitivity to tuberculin in man. Proc. Soc. exp. Biol. (N.Y.) **71**, 516—522 (1949).

LAWRENCE, H. S.: Some biological and immunological properties of transfer factor. In: Ciba Foundation Symposium on Cellular Aspects of Immunity, 243—271. Boston: Little Brown 1960.

LAWRENCE, H. S.: Transfer factor. In: Advances in Immunology **11**, 195 (1969 a).

LAWRENCE, H. S.: In: Mediators of cellular immunity. Ed.: H. S. LAWRENCE and M. LANDY. Academic Press N.Y., 145 (1969 b).

LAWRENCE, H. S., ALASKARI, S., DAVID, J. R., FRANKLIN, E. C., ZWEIMAN, B.: Transfer of immunological information in humans with dialysates of leukocytes. Trans. Ass. Amer. Phys. **76**, 84 (1963).

LAWRENCE, H. S., and FISHMAN, M.: Transfer of immunity with cell-free extract. Workshop 51. Progress in Immunology. Ed.: D. B. AMOS. Academic Press N.Y., 1395 (1972).

LEVIN, A. S., SPITLER, L. E., STITES, D. P., FUDENBERG, H. H.: Wiskott-Aldrich syndrome, a genetically determined cellular immunologic deficiency: clinical and laboratory response to therapy with transfer factor. Proc. nat. Acad. Sci. (Wash.) **67**, 821 (1970).

LYON, G., GRISCELLI, C., and LEBON, P.: Endothelial intracisternal tubular inclusions in a case of chronic encephalitis associated with immunological deficiency. Neuropädiatrie **3**, 459 (1972).

MACKANESS, G. B.: The relationship of delayed hypersensitivity to acquired cellular resistance. Brit. med. Bull. **23**, 52 (1967).

MAUPIN, M.: Technique de séparation des globules blancs. II. Techniques de séparation globale des leucocytes sanguins. Rev. Hématol. **14**, 355 (1959).

PABST, H. F., and SWANSON, R.: Successful treatment of candidiasis with transfer factor. Brit. Med. J. **1972 II**, 442.

PREUD'HOMME, J. L., GRISCELLI, C., SELIGMANN, M.: Immunoglobulins on the surface of lymphocytes in fifty patients with primary immunodeficiency diseases. Clin. Immunol. and Immunopathol. (in press).

ROCKLIN, R. E., CHILGREN, R. A., HONG, R., and DAVID, J. R.: Transfer of cellular hypersensitivity in chronic mucocutaneous candidiasis monitored *in vivo* and *in vitro*. Cell. Immunol. **1**, 290 (1970).

SCHULKIND, M. L., ADLER, W. H., ALTEMEIR, W. A., and AYOUB, E. M.: Transfer factor in the treatment of a case of chronic mucocutaneous candidiasis. Cell. Immunol. **3**, 606 (1972).

SøBORG, M.: The leukocyte migration technique for *in vitro* detection of cellular hypersensitivity in man. In: *In Vitro* Methods in Cell-Mediated Immunity. Ed.: B. R. BLOOM and P. R. GLADE. Academic Press N.Y., 297 (1971).

SPITLER, L. E., LEVIN, A. S., FUDENBERG, H. H., and HUBER, H.: Prediction of results of transfer factor therapy in the Wiskott-Aldrich syndrome by monocyte IgG receptors. Preliminary report. Sixth Leukocyte Culture Conference. Ed.: R. SCHWARZ. Academic Press N.Y., 795—800 (1972 a).

SPITLER, L. E., LEVIN, A. S., STITES, D. *et al.:* Transfer factor therapy in mucocutaneous candidiasis. Sixth Leukocyte Culture Conference 1971 (abstract).

SPITLER, L. E., LEVIN, A., STITES, D. P., FUDENBERG, H. H. *et al.:* The Wiskott-Aldrich syndrome. — Results of transfer factor therapy. J. clin. Invest. **51**, 3216 (1972 b).

TOURAINE, J. L., REVILLARD, J. P.: Application des tests cutanés d'hypersensibilité retardée à l'étude des déficits de l'immunité cellulaire. Lyon Med. **224**, 67 (1970).

TOURAINE, J. L., FREYCON, F., BETUEL, H. *et al.:* Candidose cutanéo-muqueuse chronique. Étude clinique et immunologique d'une observation et essai de traitement par le facteur de transfert. Pédiatrie (in press).

VALDIMARSSON, H., WOOD, C. B. S., HOBBS, J. R., and HOLT, P. J. L.: Immunological features in a case of chronic granulomatous candidiasis and its treatment with transfer factor. Clin. exp. Immunol. **11**, 151 (1972).

VALENTINE, F. T., and LAWRENCE, H. S.: Cell-mediated immunity. In: Advanc. intern. Med. **17**, 51—93 (1971).

Reconstitution of Cellular Immunity in Hodgkin's Disease with Transfer Factor

A. KHAN, J. M. HILL, E. LOEB, A. MACLELLAN, and N. O. HILL

Department of Immunotherapy, Leland Fikes Research Institute,
A Division of Wadley Institutes of Molecular Medicine, Dallas, TX

It has been shown by different techniques that there is impaired delayed hypersensitivity in patients with Hodgkin's disease (STEINER, 1934; DUBIN, 1947; SCHIER *et al.*, 1956; and CHASE, 1966). This is especially true in patients with active disease (AISENBERG, 1962; FAZIO *et al.*, 1962). It has also been shown that the anergic state may have definite relationship with the prognosis of the patient (SOKAL and AUNGST, 1969). Attempts have been made in the past to establish delayed hypersensitivity to tuberculin by BCG vaccination with partial success (SOKAL and AUNGST, 1969; DEMARVAL, 1940). On the other hand, passive transfer of tuberculin hypersensitivity with the aid of leukocytes had given disappointing results (KELLY *et al.*, 1960; FAZIO and CALCIATI, 1962; and MUFTUOGLO and BALKUV, 1967).

Materials and Methods

The present studies were undertaken on 11 patients who had achieved remission with radiotherapy or chemotherapy or a combination of the two, after obtaining proper consent. Instead of leukocytes, transfer factor prepared from the normal contacts of the patient was given repeatedly to 6 patients. Five patients were observed as controls. Transfer factor prepared from contacts may have an added advantage against the disease, that is, if the disease has viral etiology. The aims of this study were as follows:

1. Can large doses of transfer factor be given safely?
2. Can delayed hypersensitivity be transferred passively with repeated administration of transfer factor in Hodgkin's disease: Is transfer factor specific?
3. Can cellular immunity be reconstituted with transfer factor prepared from normal contact of the patient?
4. Can normal transfer factor prolong remission in Hodgkin's disease?

The present preliminary report will cover the first 3 points which are of interest from immunologic point of view. Patients who had gone into remission following treatment, were tested with a panel of skin test antigens. The skin tests were done 4 weeks to 27 months after the cessation of radiotherapy or chemotherapy. Normal contacts of the patients were also skin tested. The individual with maximum delayed hypersensitivity response was chosen for collection of lymphocytes. This was done with the aid of a continuous flow centrifuge (Celltrifuge-Aminco). The procedure of leukophoresis lasted for 4 hours on the average. The yield of leukozytes varied from 4.2×10^9 to 9.1×10^9 with an average of 6.6×10^9 leukozytes per donor.

Transfer factor was prepared according to the method described previously (KHAN *et al.*, 1973). Lymphocytes were ruptured by freezing and thawing. The dialyzable transfer factor was collected, lyophilized, and reconstituted to give a final concentration in which 1 ml of preparation contained transfer factor representing 10^8 leukozytes. The transfer factor was given intramuscularly in doses ranging from 1—5 ml in one injection. The interval between injections varied from daily to as far apart as 3 months. The maximum total volume of transfer factor given to a patient was 41 ml, administered in divided doses, over a period of 15 months. This represented 4.1×10^9 leukozytes. No side effects attributable to transfer factor were observed either clinically or by laboratory tests.

Results and Discussion

Table 1 shows the results of this treatment in patient R. E. The histologic diagnosis of the patient and stage of the disease is given in the left upper corner of the table. She had had BCG vaccination in the past under a different protocol. Her skin tests were still negative 27 months after the initial radiotherapy. 2 weeks after the last injection of 3 ml transfer factor, skin tests showed marked reactions to mumps, PPD and a 24 hour reaction to dermatophytin. It is interesting that the PPD reaction also became positive. The donor was negative to PPD. Therefore, even her own dormant delayed reactivity improved. In-spite of the continued treatment, her tuberculin reactivity began to subside while the passive reactivity persisted. The disease relapsed 11 months after the onset of transfer factor treatment. She received radiation to the neck and mediastinum and on the last day of radiation she again became positive to tuberculin. She received 4 courses of MVPP (nitrogen mustard, vinblastin, procarbazine and prednisolone) following radiotherapy. It is interesting that by this time the donor reactions had disappeared but weak tuberculin reaction still persisted.

Patient J. K. with mixed cellularity, stage II A disease, had a donor that reacted to all the antigens; although PPD reaction was very weak (Table 2). Most of these reactions were transferred to the recipient. She is still free from disease and has been on immunotherapy for 18 months.

Table 3 depicts a patient (L. C.) with nodular sclerosing disease. She had some reactions to the antigens to which the donor was also positive. PPD, which was weak positive in the donor, could not be transferred. This patient was not considered as positive for passive transfer. You may note that the patient did become DNCB (di-nitrochlorobenzene) positive. She has been receiving transfer factor for 15 months and she is still in remission.

J. T. also had nodular sclerosing disease, stage II A (Table 4). All the skin tests were negative 4 weeks after chemotherapy. The donor had fairly good reactions and all of them were transferred passively to the recipient. The patient is still in remission and has been on immunotherapy for 4 months.

C. J. had nodular sclerosing disease, stage III AS (Table 5). His skin tests were negative before transfer factor. Weak transfers were achieved following the administration of transfer factor. In-spite of continued administration of transfer factor for 16 months, the patient's skin tests became negative. The patient died of bronchopneumonia. An autopsy was refused. There was no clinical evidence of recurrence.

Table 1

Patient: R. E.
Histologic diagnosis: Nodular sclerosing, stage I A
Prior treatment: Radiotherapy 3500 R, BCG vaccination two years before immunotherapy

Antigen		Donor reactions mm	Recipient reactions/mm						
				After transfer factor [a]				Last day of radiation	14 days after MVPP×4
			Before	2 weeks	Imd. [b]	5 weeks			
Mumps	24 hrs.	23	—	15	16	40	Relapse	40	—
	48 hrs.	35	—	27	24	60		30	—
Histo-plasmin	24 hrs.	—	—	—	—	—		—	—
	48 hrs.	—	—	—	—	—		35	—
							Radiation 3000 R		
PPD	24 hrs.	—	—	30	—	—		23	5
	48 hrs.	—	—	30	33	—		20	5
Dermato-phytin	24 hrs.	35	—	20	9	45		—	—
	48 hrs.	—	—	—	11	—		—	—
DNCB		+	—	—	+	+		+	+
Dose of transfer factor				3 ml (Divided doses)	17 ml	5 ml			

[a] Time period denotes the interval between skin test and prior dose of transfer factor.
[b] Immediate.

The sixth patient had the disease diagnosed as mixed cellular type (Table 6). It was staged as IV A. All the skin reactions were negative. Passive transfer could not be achieved following 2 doses of 5 ml transfer factor.

2 patients also showed improved lymphocyte blastogenesis response after transfer factor. No such changes were observed in the controls.

In conclusion, passive transfer was achieved with repeated doses of transfer factor in 4 patients ranging in the stage of the disease from I A to III A. S. 1 patient with stage II A and one with IV A did not achieve passive transfer. Evidence of improved immunity was seen by the appearance of delayed hypersensitivity, DNCB reaction, or improved blastogenesis in 5 out of 6 patients. Delayed hypersensitivity appeared in the recipient which was absent in the donor. This suggests a non-specific

Table 2

Patient: J. K.
Histologic diagnosis: Mixed cellularity, stage II A
Prior treatment: MVPP × 6

Antigen		Donor reactions mm	Recipient reactions/mm			
			Before	After transfer factor [a]		
				3 weeks	2 weeks	12 weeks
Mumps	24 hrs.	25	—	5	—	4
	48 hrs.	16	—	—	—	5
Histoplasmin	24 hrs.	9	—	—	17	26
	48 hrs.	9	—	—	17	17
PPD	24 hrs.	5	—	—	—	22
	48 hrs.	—	—	—	—	—
Dermatophytin	24 hrs.	8	—	12	15	4
	48 hrs.	—	—	15	16	3
DNCB				—	—	—
Dose of transfer factor				5 ml	8 ml	8 ml
				(Divided doses)		

[a] Time period denotes the interval between skin test and prior dose of transfer factor.

Table 3

Patient: L. C
Histologic diagnosis: Nodular sclerosing, stage II A
Prior treatment: Radiation 4000 R

Antigen		Donor reactions mm	Recipient reactions/mm			
			Before	After transfer factor [a]		
				2 weeks	3 weeks	3—1/2 months
Mumps	24 hrs.	10	5	15	20	20
	48 hrs.	20	10	7	—	20
Histoplasmin	24 hrs.	—	—	—	—	—
	48 hrs.	—	—	—	—	—
PPD	24 hrs.	5	—	—	—	—
	48 hrs.	—	—	—	—	—
Dermatophytin	24 hrs.	10	—	15	—	—
	48 hrs.	12	7	—	—	—
DNCB		+		—	—	+
Dose of transfer factor				8 ml	10 ml	4 ml
				(Divided doses)		

[a] Time period denotes the interval between skin test and prior dose of transfer factor.

Table 4

Patient: J. T.
Histologic diagnosis: Nodular sclerosing, stage II A
Prior treatment: MVPP × 6

Antigen		Donor reactions mm	Recipient reactions/mm			
			Before	After transfer factor [a]		
				4 days	8 days	10 weeks
Mumps	24 hrs.	22	—	—	10	5
	48 hrs.	25	—	—	10	6
Histoplasmin	24 hrs.	10	—	15	15	15
	48 hrs.	10	—	23	16	20
PPD	24 hrs.	—	—	—	—	—
	48 hrs.	—	—	—	—	—
Dermatophytin	24 hrs.	10	—	—	—	13
	48 hrs.	—	—	—	—	15
Varidase	24 hrs.	15	—	30	22	13
	48 hrs.	20	—	20	—	—
DNCB			—	+	+	+
Dose of transfer factor				5 ml	5 ml	5 ml

[a] Time period denotes the interval between skin test and prior dose of transfer factor.

Table 5

Patient: C. J.
Histologic diagnosis: Nodular sclerosing, stage III A.S.
Prior treatment: MVPP × 6

Antigen		Donor reactions mm	Recipient reactions/mm			
			Before	After transfer factor [a]		
				Imd. [b]	4 weeks	6 weeks
Mumps	24 hrs.	20	—	8	—	—
	48 hrs.	40	—	—	—	—
Histoplasmin	24 hrs.	10	—	—	6	—
	48 hrs.	—	—	—	6	—
PPD	24 hrs.	—	—	—	—	—
	48 hrs.	—	—	—	—	—
Dermatophytin	24 hrs.	10	—	6	—	—
	48 hrs.	—	—	—	—	—
Dose of transfer factor				19 ml (Divided doses)	10 ml	10 ml

[a] Time period denotes the interval between skin test and prior dose of transfer factor.
[b] Immediate.

Table 6

Patient: T. W.
Histologic diagnosis: Mixed cellularity, stage IV A
Prior treatment: MVPP × 2, Radiation 3000 R

Antigen		Donor reactions	Recipient reactions/mm Before	After transfer factor[a]	
		mm		3 days	4 days
Mumps	24 hrs.	29	—	—	3
	48 hrs.	22	—	—	3
Histoplasmin	24 hrs.	—	—	—	—
	48 hrs.	—	—	—	—
PPD	24 hrs.	—	—	—	—
	48 hrs.	—	—	—	—
Dermatophytin	24 hrs.	26	—	—	—
	48 hrs.	35	—	—	—
Varidase	24 hrs.	—	—	—	—
	48 hrs.	—	—	—	—
DNCB			+	+	+
Dose of transfer factor				5 ml	5 ml

[a] Time period denotes the interval between skin test and prior dose of transfer factor.

effect of the transfer factor in addition to the specific transfer of the donor reactivity. This may be explained on the basis of non-specificity of the factor or the presence of multiple factors in the dialyzable fraction. The later may be more appropriate since specific transfer of activity was also observed. Side effects attributable to transfer factor were not seen.

Acknowledgments

We thank Simone Thaxton for her technical assistance in conducting the immune studies on the patients and in the preparation of transfer factor.

References

AISENBERG, A. C.: Studies on delayed hypersensitivity in Hodgkin's disease. J. clin. Invest. **41,** 1964 (1962).

CHASE, M. W.: Delayed-type hypersensitivity and the immunology of Hodgkin's disease, with a parallel examination of sarcoidosis. Cancer Res. **26,** 1097 (1966).

DEMARVAL, L.: Los pacientes afectados de limifogranulomatosis maligna son insensibles a dosis masivas de tuberculina bruta inyectida por via subcutanea. Pren. méd. argent. **27,** 2310 (1940).

DUBIN, I. N.: The poverty of the immunological mechanism in patients with Hodgkin's disease. Ann. intern. Med. **27,** 898 (1947).

Fazio, M., Calciati, A.: An attempt to transfer tuberculin hypersensitivity in Hodgkin's disease. Panminerva med. 4, 164 (1962).
Fazio, M., Calciati, A., Depaoli, M.: Dermatite allergica de contatto nel linfogranuloma maligno. Minerva derm. 37, 259 (1962).
Kelly, W. D., Lamb, D. L., Varco, R. L., Good, R. A.: An investigation of Hodgkin's disease with respect to the problem of homotransplantation. Ann. N.Y. Acad. Sci. 87, 187 (1960).
Khan, A., Hill, J. M., Loeb, E., Maclellan, A., Hill, N. O.: Management of Chediak-Higashi syndrome with transfer factor. Amer. J. Dis. Child. In press (1973).
Muftuoglo, A. U., Balkuv, S.: Passive transfer of tuberculin sensitivity to patients with Hodgkin's disease. New Engl. J. Med. 277, 126 (1967).
Schier, W. W., Roth, A., Ostroff, G., Schrift, M. J.: Hodgkin's disease and immunity. Amer. J. Med. 20, 94 (1956).
Sokal, J. D., Aungst, C. W.: Response to BCG vaccination and survival in advanced Hodgkin's disease. Cancer (Philad.) 24, 128 (1969).
Steiner, P. E.: Etiology of Hodgkin's disease; skin reactions to avian and human tuberculin proteins in Hodgkin's disease. Arch. intern. Med. 54, 11 (1934).

Complications of Cancer Chemotherapy. The Special Case of Hormones*

J. C. HEUSON

Service de Médecine et d'Investigation Clinique de l'Institut J. Bordet, Bruxelles

Side effects of hormones given for the treatment of neoplastic diseases, such as for example breast cancer, depend upon mechanisms quite different from those operating with other chemotherapeutic agents. This is precisely because hormones are usually not cytotoxic and that their antitumor efficacy appears to be based more on regulatory mechanisms than on cytotoxicity.

Side effects of hormones belong to three main categories (Table 1). Firstly they may result from the use of hormones at supraphysiological doses or of hormones of the opposite sex. Secondly, side effects may occasionally be due to non-hormonal

Table 1. Complications of cancer chemotherapy. The special case of hormones

Side effects due to:
1. Supraphysiological doses of hormones
2. Non-hormonal toxicity of synthetic compounds
3. Stimulation of tumor growth

toxicity of synthetic compounds. Thirdly, and this is the most interesting, complications may sometimes result from stimulation of tumor growth and exacerbation of the disease by hormones which usually achieve the opposite, namely beneficial effect. This type of complication is of particular interest because 1. it does not occur with other types of chemotherapy, 2. it is related to the very mechanism of the anti-tumor action of hormones, and 3. it makes the use of hormones in cancer a more difficult task than is usually thought and imposes on the clinician to be especially alert when treating his patients. Not only can hormones be inactive in a given person, just as it happens with cytotoxic compounds, but they may actually aggravate the disease by enhancing tumor growth, which other drugs usually do not. Indeed, one exception may exist in relation to the immunodepressive effect of cytotoxic drugs, but then the mechanism is indirect and different.

* Part of this work was supported by a grant from the "Fonds Cancérologique de la Caisse Générale d'Epargne et de Retraite de Belgique" and performed within the framework of the Association Euratom, University of Brussels and University of Pisa.

The first category of side effects results from the use of hormones at supraphysiological doses, or of hormones of the opposite sex. This topic will only be briefly discussed because it is concerned with well-known effects. The more important are listed in Table 2. One special consideration about androgens: much effort has been devoted to suppress their virilizing effects by synthesizing new derivatives. Partial decrease was obtained with drugs such as Durabolin (FORD, 1959) and more recently Drostanolone (PETIT *et al.*, 1971), also called Masteril (HELMAN and BENNETT, 1972). Nevertheless, these compounds retain considerable virilizing activity. More complete success was achieved with Δ_1-testololactone (GOLDENBERG *et al.*, 1973) and 7β-17α-dimethyl-testosterone (Calusterone) (GORDAN *et al.*, 1972 and GOLDENBERG *et al.*, 1973). The former is completely devoid of androgenicity; the latter seems almost free of this property although, among androgen derivatives, it appears to be one of the most effective in the treatment of breast cancer.

Table 2. Hormonal side effects due to supraphysiological dosage

1. *Androgens*	virilization, hoarseness, increased libido
Non-virilizing derivatives[a]:	
	Δ_1-testololactone (18% remission rate)
	7β,17α-dimethyltestosterone (28% remission rate).
2. *Estrogens*	anorexia, nausea, vomiting, sodium and water retention, uterine bleeding, pigmentation of skin, increased libido, vascular thrombosis
3. *Progestogens*	nausea, vomiting
4. *Corticosteroids*	Cushingoid appearance, hyperglycemia, peptic ulcers, immunodepression

[a] GOLDENBERG, WATERS, RAVDIN, ANSFIELD and SEGALOFF (1973).

The second type of side effects is concerned with non-hormonal toxicity of synthetic compounds (Table 3). Induction of hepatic dysfunction is characteristic of the methyl derivatives of testosterone. It seems much less frequent with the dimethyltestosterone compound Calusterone already quoted (GORDAN *et al.*, 1972 and GOLDENBERG *et al.*, 1973). The anti-estrogen Nafoxidine, at the dosage of 60 mg three times a day, induces phototoxicity and variable degrees of dryness of the skin and loss of hair (HEUSON *et al.*, 1972). Lowering the doses 6 times completely or almost completely abolishes these side effects (personal observation), but the therapeutic efficacy at this lower dosage has yet to be established. Tamoxifen, another anti-estrogen active at a dose of 20 to 40 mg daily, often produces hot flushes and sometimes mild thrombocytopenia (COLE *et al.*, 1971).

Table 3. Non-hormonal toxicity of synthetic compounds

1. Methyl and dimethyltestosterone: hepatic dysfunction
2. Nafoxidine: dryness of skin, loss of hair, phototoxicity
3. Tamoxifen: hot flushes, thrombocytopenia

The third class of complications consists of hormonally-induced exacerbation of advanced breast cancer. Hypercalcemia, which is often quickly lethal, is representative of this category. Fig. 1 depicts the clinical course of a patient who died from this complication. It is significant that two hormones with supposedly opposite or antagonistic effects, namely an estrogen and an androgen, both produced acute episodes of hypercalcemia. The mechanism of this complication is unknown, but is

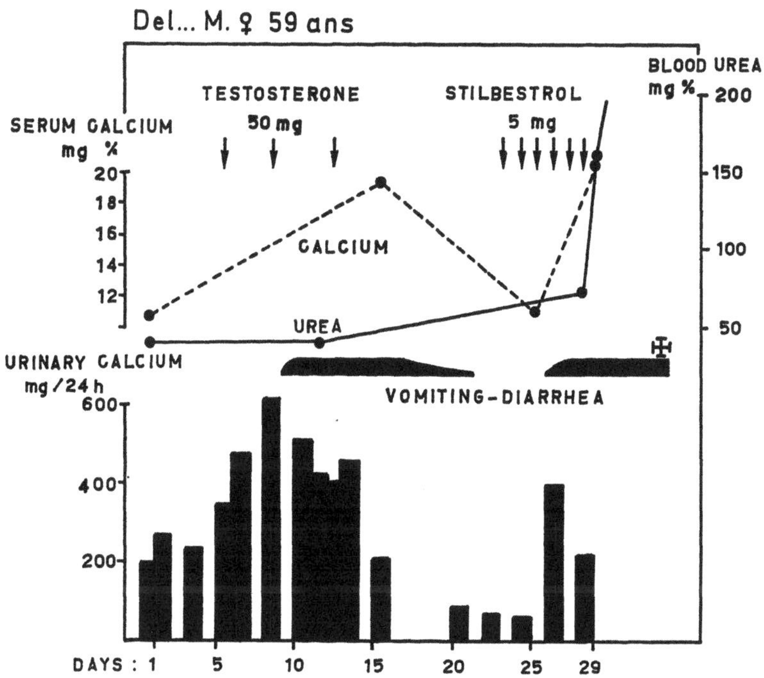

Fig. 1. Hypercalcemia and hypercalciuria induced in a case of breast cancer metastatic to bones by both estrogenic and androgenic treatments (H. J. Tagnon, unpublished)

usually explained by an enhancement of tumor growth (Pearson *et al.*, 1954; Karhausen *et al.*, 1955). A change in the metabolic activity of the tumor cells could also be incriminated. It should be stressed that besides hypercalcemia, aggravation may consist of sudden increase in respiratory distress, compression of vital organs, etc.

An interesting question is why both estrogens and androgens may have the same enhancing effect even in a same patient. One possible explanation is that the androgens are transformed into estrogens in various tissues, particularly in adipose tissue. It will be seen that other hormonally-related compounds may also induce hypercalcemia.

Ascribing to the estrogens the stimulating role does not actually imply that it is by a direct effect. Thus, it has been claimed that prolactin might enhance breast cancer growth in some patients. This contention is primarily based on the observation of the beneficial effect of hypophysectomy and by the demonstration that, in the rat mammary tumor model, prolactin is the hormone involved (Pearson *et al.*, 1969). This problem has been thoroughly discussed elsewhere (Heuson, 1974).

We have therefore studied in a few postmenopausal women the effect of therapeutic doses of estrogens on prolactin secretion. The results presented in Table 4 clearly demonstrate that estrogens markedly increase the blood prolactin levels. These data are consistent with the view that estrogen-induced hypercalcemia could result from stimulation of prolactin secretion.

Table 4. Effect of oral ethinylestradiol (EO, 3 mg daily) on serum prolactin level (mU/ml) [a]

Subject	Before EO		After EO		Stat. sign. [b]
	N° determinations	Mean ± s.e.	N° determinations	Mean ± s.e.	
G. E.	9	573 ±55	6	946 ±138	$p < 0.025$
DK. C.	6	427 ±26	5	1,067 ±123	$p < 0.01$
DS. M.	5	90 ± 3	7	210 ± 25	$p < 0.01$

[a] L'Hermite, Heuson and Robyn.
[b] Student's *t* test.

This possibility led us to think that compounds active on breast cancer but devoid of prolactin stimulating activity might not produce such complications and by the same token possibility be more effective than estrogens in the treatment of breast cancer. We therefore studied the effect of Nafoxidine on prolactin secretion. Nafoxidine is a compound which behaves mainly as a potent antiestrogen although it has weak estrogenic properties (Gallez *et al.*, 1973). It has been shown active on breast cancer by the EORTC Breast Cancer Cooperative Group (Heuson *et al.*, 1972). The data presented in Table 5 show that Nafoxidine did not stimulate prolactin secretion and even was inhibitor in one patient. And yet, it was reported by a member of the EORTC Breast Cancer Cooperative Group to have induced hypercalcemia in one patient. This would indicate that stimulation of prolactin secretion may not be the mechanism or the only mechanism involved, but that a direct effect of hormones may be responsible. In the case of Nafoxidine, induction of hypercalcemia could possibly be due to its weak estrogenic properties and resultant stimulation of tumor growth in some patients.

The hypothesis of a direct enhancing effect of Nafoxidine on mammary tumor growth was studied in the DMBA-induced mammary tumors of the rats, which we use as a model for the hormone-dependent human breast cancer. In the experiment of Fig. 2, Nafoxidine was given to tumor-bearing rats. It produced an obvious and significant inhibition of tumor growth. However, despite the average significant inhibition of growth, we did not observe the dramatic and near-complete regression which follows ovariectomy in these animals. Instead, some tumors decreased in size but others kept slowly growing. There were two possible explanations to this difference between Nafoxidine administration and ovariectomy. Either Nafoxidine antagonizes only partly the effect of the endogenous estrogens; or, it has some stimulating effect of its own on tumor growth.

To test the latter hypothesis, we subjected tumor-bearing rats to ovariectomy. They were then randomly allocated to two groups, a control group and one receiving Nafoxidine at the same dosage as in the previous experiment. The results are

Table 5. Effect of oral Nafoxidine (180 mg daily) on serum prolactin level (mU/ml) [a]

Subject	Before Nafoxidine		After Nafoxidine		Stat. sign. [b]
	N° determinations	Mean ± s.e.	N° determinations	Mean ± s.e.	
V. E.	6	166 ±28	3	218 ±73	n. s.
A. D.	6	480 ±11	5	321 ±22	$p < 0.01$
G. E.	3	111 ±69	5	59 ±15	n. s.
M. I.	4	50 ±10	4	67 ±12	n. s.

[a] L'Hermite, Heuson and Robyn.
[b] Student's t test.

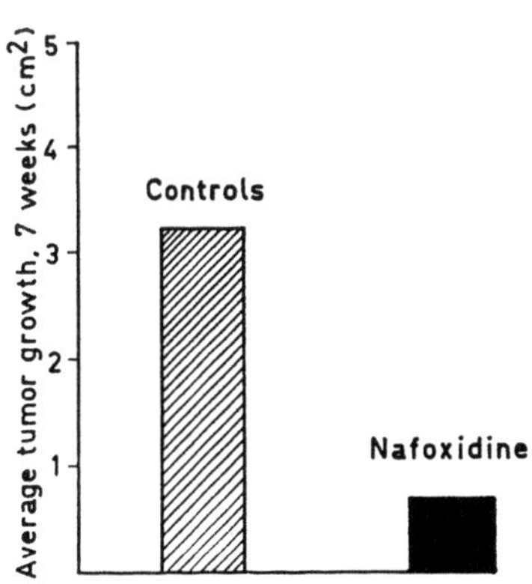

Fig. 2. Inhibitory effect of Nafoxidine on growth of the DMBA-induced rat mammary tumors (Heuson *et al.*, 1971/1972)

shown in Fig. 3. As expected, there was a near-complete regression of the tumors after ovariectomy. In contrast, under Nafoxidine administration, there was hardly a 50% reduction in mean tumor surface per rat. There were even a few tumors which continued to grow and a few which were newly formed. This indicates that Nafoxidine, besides its inhibitory effect due to its antiestrogenic properties has some stimulating effect of its own on mammary tumor growth.

In regard to human breast cancer, Nafoxidine undoubtedly has a potent therapeutic activity. Preliminary results of a comparative trial of the EORTC Breast Cancer Cooperative Group (unpublished) suggest that this activity might be greater than that of ethinylestradiol. Nevertheless, the possibility that Nafoxidine may stimulate tumor growth in some patients should be kept in mind by the clinicians concerned. Another consequence is that the search should continue for new compounds active in breast cancer and devoid of growth-stimulating activity accounting for therapeutic failures and complications of the kind discussed today, such as hypercalcemia, aggravation of respiratory distress, and others.

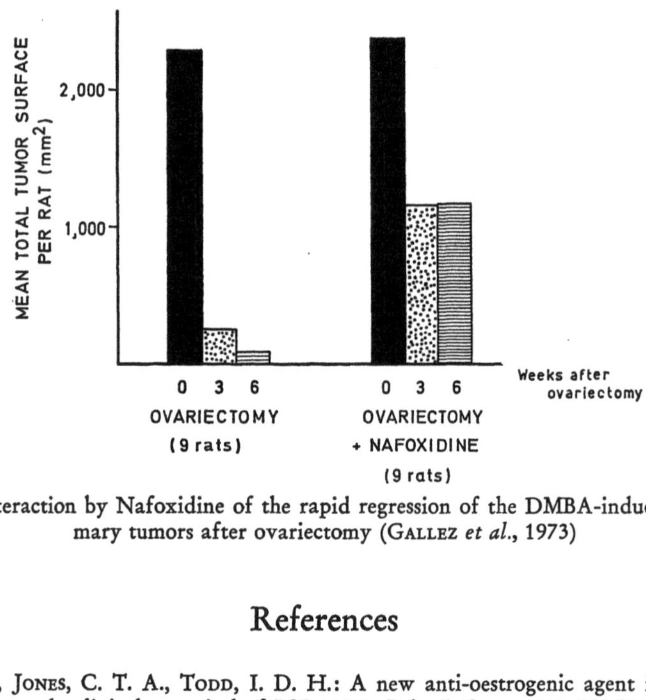

Fig. 3. Counteraction by Nafoxidine of the rapid regression of the DMBA-induced rat mammary tumors after ovariectomy (GALLEZ *et al.*, 1973)

References

COLE, M. P., JONES, C. T. A., TODD, I. D. H.: A new anti-oestrogenic agent in late breast cancer. An early clinical appraisal of ICI 46474. Brit. J. Cancer **25**, 270 (1971).

FORD, H. T.: Durabolin and Deca-Durabolin in the treatment of advanced mammary cancer. A. R. Brit. Emp. Cancer Campgn **37**, 267 (1959).

GALLEZ, GH., HEUSON, J. C., WAELBROECK, CH.: Growth-stimulating effect of Nafoxidine on rat mammary tumor after ovariectomy. Europ. J. Cancer **9**, 699 (1973).

GOLDENBERG, I. S., WATERS, M. N., RAVDIN, R. S., ANSFIELD, F. J., SEGALOFF, A.: Cooperative Breast Cancer Group: Androgenic therapy for advanced breast cancer in women. J. Amer. med. Ass. **223**, 1267 (1973).

GORDAN, G. S., WESSLER, S., AVIOLI, L. V.: Calusterone in the therapy for advanced breast cancer. J. Amer. med. Ass. **219**, 483 (1972).

HELMAN, P., BENNETT, M. B.: Hormone therapy of breast cancer with special reference to Masteril therapy. S. Afr. med. J. **46**, 1195 (1972).

HEUSON, J. C., COUNE, A., STAQUET, M.: European Breast Cancer Group: Clinical trial of Nafoxidine (U-11.100 A) in advanced breast cancer. Europ. J. Cancer **8**, 387 (1972).

HEUSON, J. C., WAELBROECK, CH., LEGROS, N., GALLEZ, GH., ROBYN, C., L'HERMITE, M.: Inhibition of DMBA-induced mammary carcinogenesis in the rat by 2-Br-α-ergocryptine (CB 154), an inhibitor of prolactin secretion, and by Nafoxidine (U-11,100 A), an estrogen antagonist. Hormones and Antagonists. Gynec. Invest. **2**, 130 (1971/72).

HEUSON, J. C.: The role of prolactin inhibition in the treatment of advanced breast cancer. Mammary Cancer and Neuroendocrine Therapy. B. STOLL, Ed. p. 349. London: Butterworths 1974.
KARHAUSEN, L., KENIS, Y., SMULDERS, J., PARMENTIER, R.: Hypercalcémie et néphrocalcinose. Etude de quartre cas de cancer du sein avec métastases osseuses. Acta clin. belg. X, 295 (1955).
L'HERMITE, M., HEUSON, J. C., ROBYN, CL.: Unpublished data.
PEARSON, O. H., WEST, C. D., HOLLANDER, V. P., TREVES, N. E.: Evaluation of endocrine therapy for advanced breast cancer. J. Amer. med. Ass. **154,** 234 (1954).
PEARSON, O. H., LLERENA, O., LLERENA, L., MOLINA, A., BUTLER, T.: Prolactin-dependent rat mammary cancer: a model for man? Trans. Ass. Amer. Phycns **82,** 225 (1969).
PETIT, J. C., KLEIN, TH., RODIER, D.: Traitement hormonal du cancer du sein avancé par le propionate de drostanolone. Bull. Cancer **58,** 511 (1971).

Factors Modifying the Activity and Toxicity of Anticancer Agents

F. SPREAFICO, M. G. DONELLI, A. VECCHI, A. BOSSI, and S. GARATTINI

Istituto di Ricerche Farmacologiche „Mario Negri", Milano

It is a common experience in cancer chemotherapy, as in practically every other field of therapeutics, that the response to treatment with antineoplastic agents quite frequently varies between individuals. Variability in therapeutic effectiveness can depend on the tumor itself and on the host; our knowledge of both these aspects is still quite limited, especially at the clinical level. In this paper we concentrate mainly on the host's contribution to variability, using experimental models to study factors which, at different levels, may decisively influence the chemotherapeutic efficacy and toxicity of anticancer agents.

A first factor which may play a role is the genetic constitution of the tumor-bearing host; this may influence, for instance, various aspects of the metabolism of exogenous compounds and consequently their bioavailability. Table 1 shows that the same dose of cyclophosphamide (cyclo-P) injected in CD_1 or CDF_1 (Balb/c $\times$ DBA/2) mice gives quite different *in vivo* effects, since in the F_1 hybrid mice greater leukopenia was observed as well as increased immunosuppressive activity, as revealed by the lower numbers in the spleen of anti-sheep erythrocyte hemolytic plaque-forming cells (PFC) detectable with the technique of JERNE and NORDIN (1963). This difference in cytotoxic activity is attributable to a higher capacity of CDF_1 mice to activate the drug; in fact, cyclo-P itself is cytotoxically inactive and must be processed by the microsomal system (mainly of the liver) to active metabolite(s) (BROCK and HOHORST, 1967; CONNORS *et al.*, 1970; HILL *et al.*, 1972; SLADEK, 1973). The CDF_1 mice display a significantly higher plasma level of cyclo-P-derived alkylating activity, measurable with the procedure described by FRIEDMAN and BOGER (1961) early after drug injection and a much longer duration of this activity. *In vitro,* liver microsomal preparations of CDF_1 mice after incubation with cyclo-P give rise to more alkylating activity and faster than similar preparations from CD_1 mice.

Circadian rhythmicity is another often neglected factor which can give different drug concentrations in the body and thus result in variable responses *in vivo.*

Possibly the best known example of this daily rhythmicity concerns the metabolism of steroids; a dose of hydrocortisone (1.5 mg/kg i.v.) injected in man at 8 a.m. gave a plasma half-life of 107 ± 11 min; the same dose administered at 4 p.m. gave a value of only 73 ± 8 min (MORSELLI *et al.*, 1970 a). This phenomenon is not restricted to steroids but can be observed with other frequently employed antitumor drugs, as illustrated in Table 2 for 6-mercaptopurine (6-MP). The same table also shows the potential importance of another factor in controlling drug levels in the body and therefore antitumor activity and toxicity, since the daily rhythmicity in 6-MP metabolism is present only in female rats. A further example of the possible influence of sex in influencing variability of response through a different metabolic

Table 1. *In vivo* activity and metabolic parameters of cyclophosphamide (50 mg/kg i.v.) in CD_1 and (Balb/c × DBA/2)F_1 hybrid mice

	(Balb/c × DBA/2)F_1	CD_1
Leukopenic activity (% of controls)	43 ± 7	73 ± 2 [a]
Immunosuppressive activity (PFC/spleen)	765 ± 312	4,280 ± 545 [a]
Volume of distribution (l/kg ± 95% confid. limits)	0.30 ± 0.04	0.22 ± 0.10
T_{10} plasma alkylating activity (mμmoles HN_2-equiv./ml ± S.E.)	153 ± 10	118 ± 7 [a]
T_{60} plasma alkylating activity) (mμmoles HN_2-equiv./ml ± S.E.)	60.9 ± 3.2	34.7 ± 3.6 [a]
$T^{1/2}$ plasma alkylating activity (min ± 95% confid. limits)	50 ± 8	20 ± 2 [a]
In vitro microsomal metabolism (mμmoles HN_2-equiv./g liver ± S.E.)	911.6 ± 12.7	695.2 ± 39.1 [a]

[a] $p < 0.05$.

Table 2. Influence of time of injection on 6-mercaptopurine (50 mg/kg i.v.) peak serum levels in Sprague Dawley rats

Time of injection	peak serum levels (μg/ml ± S.E.)	
	males	females
9.00 a.m.	81 ± 6	50 ± 5
9.00 p.m.	90 ± 1	99 ± 6 [a]

[a] $p < 0.05$.

capacity may be seen in the marked differences in 6-MP levels in male and female rats of the same strain given an equal dose of drug at the same hour of the day.

The age of the host can be very important in influencing the effectiveness of any therapy. Table 3 shows that differences due to age may not depend only on a different susceptibility to and capacity of recovery from toxicity but also on a difference in capacity to eliminate the administered compounds.

Another factor which may markedly modify the activity of antineoplastic agents is additional medication given earlier or concomitantly to the tumor-bearing host.

Table 3. Serum levels of 6-mercaptopurine (50 mg/kg i.v.) in Sprague Dawley rats of different ages

Age (days)	6-MP (μg/ml) after min			T ½ (min)
	1	5	30	
21	77	30	11	12.1
50	71	23	6.7 [a]	9.0
75	75	10 [a]	2.9 [a]	6.2 [a]

[a] $p < 0.05$.

Table 4. Plasma levels of methotrexate (500 mg/kg) after oral administration in mice pretreated with cyclophosphamide (300 mg/kg i.p.) 1 or 7 days earlier

Min after MTX administration	μg/ml MTX		
	Controls	cyclo-P 1 d	cyclo-P 7 d
15	5.7	11.5 [a]	13.0 [a]
30	4.1	6.1 [a]	8.5 [a]
60	3.0	6.2 [a]	6.6 [a]
240	1.4	2.1 [a]	2.3 [a]

[a] $p < 0.05$.

Table 5. Effect of cyclophosphamide (300 mg/kg i.p.) pretreatment on serum level of 6-mercaptopurine (50 mg/kg) injected intravenously 7 days later in mice

Pretreatment	μg/ml after min			T½ (min)	Vd (1/kg)
	1	15	30		
Saline	51.92 ± 2.9	16.0 ± 1.1	9.4 ± 0.3	5′24″ (4′46″—6′04″)	0.82 (0.64—1.00)
Cyclo-P	66.1 ± 3.0 [a]	27.1 ± 1.5 [a]	21.8 ± 1.5 [a]	11′20″ [a] (8′25″—14′15″)	0.91 (0.79—1.13)

[a] $p < 0.01$.

Table 6. Serum levels of daunomycin (800 mg/kg os) in mice pretreated 7 days earlier with cyclophosphamide (300 mg/kg i.p.)

Pretreatment	μg/ml after min		
	15	30	240
Saline	1.66 ± 0.1	5.53 ± 0.2	8.63 ± 0.1
Cyclo-P	5.07 ± 0.1 [a]	3.87 ± 0.1 [a]	4.83 ± 0.1 [a]

[a] $p < 0.01$.

At a time when multiple treatments are almost standard practice in cancer chemotherapy, drug interactions are particularly important. From Table 4 it can be seen that if mice have been pretreated with cyclo-P 1 or 7 days previously, subsequent oral administration of methotrexate (MTX) results in MTX blood levels that are twice as high as in controls. A second example, which does not seem to be even partly explainable by a greater degree of drug absorption through the damaged gut, as in the case presented above, is shown in Table 5. A doubling of the serum half-life of intravenously administered 6-MP is seen in mice given a single injection of cyclo-P one week earlier. In both these cases the long duration of the effects of these pretreatments is apparent. To show how complicated the picture may be, it should be noted that the same type of pretreatment will not always result in the same qualitative kind of modification of the bioavailability of subsequently administered drugs. As shown in Table 6, whereas pretreatment of mice with cyclo-P prolonged the half-life of 6-MP and MTX, reduced blood levels are seen with daunomycin. Failure of a generally appropriate dose of agent to reach its full antitumoral effect may be seen as a form of toxicity. These results emphasize once again the importance of monitoring drug levels so as to adapt the treatment to the individual patient.

Table 7. Immunodepressive activity in mice of the L-asparaginase–methotrexate combination according to the relative order of injection of the two agents

L-asparaginase I.U./mouse i.p.	Methotrexate mg/kg i.p.	PFC/spleen (× 10^3)
—	—	420
50 (day 0)	—	60 [a]
—	20 (day 1)	6 [a]
50 (day 0)	20 (day 1)	56 [a]

Methotrexate mg/kg i.p.	L-asparaginase I.U./mouse i.p.	PFC/spleen (× 10^3)
—	—	335
20 (day 0)	—	38 [a]
—	50 (day 1)	213
20 (day 0)	50 (day 1)	37 [a]

[a] $p < 0.05$. CD_1 mice were injected with 4.10^8 sheep erythrocytes i.p. on day 0; the immune response was assessed on day 4 by JERNE's technique.

With combination chemotherapy the order of drug administration should also be considered, since it may determine whether synergism or antagonism operates. Table 7 shows that, if L-asparaginase is injected in mice before MTX, the immunosuppressive effect of MTX can be abolished or very markedly reduced, i.e. when the enzyme is administered 3—24 h before the antifolic. The same schedule-dependent antagonism affects the antitumoral activity of this combination, witness the number of L 5178 Y leukemia cells present in the peritoneal cavity in the different experimental groups (Table 8). When MTX is given first, neither antagonism nor synergism is observed. A discussion of the mechanisms that could underlie these observations is presented elsewhere (SPREAFICO *et al.*, 1973 a), together with further examples of drug interaction in cytotoxic treatment. One more example is presented here, since it concerns two drugs widely used in clinical treatment: prednisone and cyclo-P (Table 9).

Table 8. Antileukemic effect of methotrexate in mice pretreated with L-asparaginase

Exp. group	No. of L 5178 Y leukemia cells ($\times 10^6$) in the peritoneal cavity at day	
	7	8
Controls	121.4	216.3
L-asparaginase	47.1	96.7
MTX	6.3	19.2
L-asparaginase + MTX	32.6 [a]	61.8 [a]

[a] $p < 0.01$. CDF_1 mice were injected with 10^5 L 5178 Y cells i.p. on day 0, and with L-asparaginase (25,000 I.U./kg i.p.) on days 1 and 2; MTX (20 mg/kg i.p.) was injected on day 2, 4 h after L-asparaginase.

Table 9. Immunosuppressive activity in mice of the prednisone–cyclophosphamide combination according to the time of injection of each drug

Treatment (mg/kg i.p.)	Day of injection	PFC/spleen (% of controls)
Predn. 50	1 or 2	100
Cyclo-P 25	2	2.3
Predn. 50 +	1	7.4 [a]
Cyclo-P 25	2	
Cyclo-P 25 +	2	0.5 [a]
Predn. 50	2	

[a] $p < 0.05$. Mice were injected on day 0 with 4.10^8 sheep erythrocytes; immune response was assessed on day 4 by JERNE's technique.

The cancer patient is frequently given not only anticancer drugs but also other types of medication (RALL, 1967) administered as general supportive treatment for additional specific medical problems. We have investigated possible interactions between antineoplastic drugs and other agents. Table 10 shows the remarkable increase in the immunosuppressive activity of 6-MP injected in mice pretreated with two doses of phenobarbital (typifying a class of agents very frequently employed in hospitals). A modification in cytotoxic activity following treatment with phenobarbital was observed for other antitumor agents. Among drugs so far tested, an increase in immunosuppressive activity has been found in mice given doses of 1,3-bis(2-chloroethyl)-1-nitrosourea (BCNU), procarbanize and triethylen-melamine, whereas a strong reduction in activity was seen for hydrocortisone and cyclo-P. To re-emphasize the possible effect of the treatment schedule on the effectiveness and

Table 10. Effect of phenobarbital pretreatment on the immunosuppressive activity of 6-mercaptopurine in mice

Exp. group	PFC/spleen
Controls	418,300
Phenobarb.	432,600
6-MP	53,750
Phenobarb. + 6-MP	16,920 [a]

[a] $p < 0.01$. Phenobarb. (80 mg/kg i.p.) was injected on days 0 and 1, 6-MP (100 mg/kg i.v.) was injected on day 2.

Table 11. Immune responsiveness in mice chronically treated with phenobarbital and given single or repeated injections of cyclophosphamide

Exp. group	Dose (mg/kg i.p.)	PFC/spleen
Controls	—	296,425
Phenobarb.	40 × 6	282,650
Cyclo-P	35 × 1	33,875
Phenobarb. + Cyclo-P	40 × 6 35 × 1	149,880 [a]
Cyclo-P	35 × 4	7,540
Phenobarb. + Cyclo-P	40 × 6 35 × 4	1,635 [a]

[a] $p < 0.01$. CDF_1 mice challenged with 4.10^8 sheep erythrocytes on day 0, were given phenobarbital from days —4 to —1; immune response was assessed by JERNE's technique on day 4.

safety of a chemotherapeutic treatment, the data presented in Table 11 may be useful. In mice pretreated with a series of injections of phenobarbital, the effect of a subsequent single dose of cyclo-P is markedly reduced in comparison with animals given only the immunosuppressant. Conversely, a marked increase in the cytotoxic activity of cyclo-P is observed when animals chronically treated with barbiturate are given, instead of single injections, a more prolonged course of cyclo-P (SPREAFICO *et al.*, 1973 b). Lastly, it should be noted that the influence of other drugs on the host's metabolic capacity relative to antitumoral compounds can be very long-lasting: in man, a marked decrease in the half-life of corticosteroids can be seen as long as 20 days after stopping barbiturate treatment (MORSELLI *et al.*, 1970 b).

In conclusion, the examples given illustrate only some of the factors which may affect the toxicity and alter the effectiveness of available antitumor treatment. It is clear that much still remains to be learned concerning the pharmacology of anticancer agents if we aim to administer rational, on-target cancer therapy.

Acknowledgement

The experimental work summarized in this paper was supported by a grant from Euratom (088-72-1-BIAC) and by contracts from NIH (NCI-C-72-3242) and CNR (72.00207.04).

References

BROCK, N., HOHORST, H.-J.: Metabolism of cyclophosphamide. Cancer (Philad.) **20**, 900 (1967).

CONNORS, T. A., GROVER, P. L., MCLOUGHLIN, A. M.: Microsomal activation of cyclophosphamide *in vivo*. Biochem. Pharmacol. **19**, 1533 (1970).

FRIEDMAN, O. N., BOGER, E.: Colorimetric estimation of nitrogen mustards in aqueous media. Hydrolytic behavior of bis(β-chloroethyl)amine, nor-HN_2. Analyt. Chem. **33**, 906 (1961).

HILL, D. L., LASTER, W. R., JR., STRUCK, R. F.: Enzymic metabolism of cyclophosphamide and nicotine and production of a toxic cyclophosphamide metabolite. Cancer Res. **32**, 658 (1972).

JERNE, N. K., NORDIN, A. A.: Plaque formation in agar by single antibody-producing cells. Science **140**, 405 (1963).

MORSELLI, P. L., MARC, V., GARATTINI, S., ZACCALA, M.: Metabolism of exogenous cortisol in humans. I. Diurnal variation in plasma disappearance rate. Biochem. Pharmacol. **19**, 1643 (1970 a).

MORSELLI, P. L., MARC, V., GARATTINI, S., ZACCALA, M.: Metabolism of exogenous cortisol in humans. Influence of phenobarbital treatment on plasma cortisol disappearance rate. Rev. Europ. Étud. clin. biol. **15**, 195 (1970 b).

RALL, D. P.: Pharmacologic aspects of selective chemotherapy of leukemia and Burkitt's tumor. Combination chemotherapy, advertent and inadvertent. Cancer Res. **27**, 2650 (1967).

SLADEK, N. E.: Bioassay and relative cytotoxic potency of cyclophosphamide metabolites generated *in vitro* and *in vivo*. Cancer Res. **33**, 1150 (1973).

SPREAFICO, F., VECCHI, A., ANACLERIO, A., MANTOVANI, A.: Drug interactions in cytotoxic treatment. Manuscript in preparation (1973 a).

SPREAFICO, F., MANTOVANI, A., ANACLERIO, A., VECCHI, A.: Negative interactions in chemical immunosuppression. In preparation (1973 b).

Modification of Drug Metabolism Induced in the Host by the Presence of a Tumor

I. Bartošek, M. G. Donelli, and A. Guaitani

Istituto di Ricerche Farmacologiche „Mario Negri", Milano

The presence of a tumor in a host results in marked changes at the levels of various organs, including the liver. A functional change in the liver metabolism may be detected by measuring the activity and the metabolism of drugs.

An example of these modifications is the significant difference in sleeping time following pentobarbital administration to Sprague Dawley rats. It was shown that rats bearing Walker 256 carcinosarcoma sleep longer (71 ± 9 min) than controls (16 ± 2 min) after receiving the same dose of the barbiturate.

The pentobarbital levels in plasma and in brain were much higher in tumor-bearing rats than in control animals (Rosso *et al.*, 1968). The activities of liver microsomal enzymes that are responsible for the hydroxylation and hence detoxification of pentobarbital were considerably decreased in tumor bearing animals (Rosso *et al.*, 1971).

In order to analyze the metabolic role of liver in the presence of a tumor the technique of isolated perfused liver was used. This technique obviates the problems encountered *in vivo*, where a drug is not only metabolized but also excreted, or bound to proteins and distributed in several tissues. It also has the advantage over *in vitro* enzyme preparations (e.g. liver microsomal enzymes) of maintaining the integrity of the liver cells.

Moreover, the conditions of liver perfusion can easily be modified, e.g. by pretreating separately the donors of the liver or of the blood for the perfusion, by changing the composition of the perfusion medium, by introducing substrates by infusion, by using dialysis, or by changing blood flow, temperature, etc.

In the perfusion apparatus utilized in this study, the liver was attached through the portal vein to a cannula and supported by a soft membrane. Samples of the perfusing medium were collected after its passage through the liver; the medium was then saturated by a gas mixture containing 95% O_2 + 5% CO_2 in a thin-film rotating oxygenator. The roller pump supplies the oxygenated medium through two containers, which also function as bubble traps before the liquid reaches the liver cannula (Fig. 1) (Bartošek *et al.*, 1972 a).

In our experiments male Sprague Dawley rats weighing 220 ± 10 g were used as donors of liver and blood. Walker 256 carcinosarcoma was transplanted subcutaneously 12 days before the animals were used as donors of blood and/or liver in the perfusion experiments. The average weight of liver of normal rats was 10.3 ± 0.4 g and that of tumor-bearing animals 12.0 ± 0.4 g. The average weight of Walker tumors was 32.9 ± 1.6 g.

The perfusion medium was 1/3 heparinized and defibrinated rat blood, 1/3 homologous serum and 1/3 Krebs-Ringer bicarbonate buffer at pH 7.4. The drugs under study were added to the perfusion medium in concentrations of from 20—150 μg/ml. The liver was perfused by recirculation; the flow of the medium was 1 ml min^{-1} g^{-1} of liver. The total volume of medium used was proportional to the weight of the liver (5 ml of medium to 1 g of hepatic tissue).

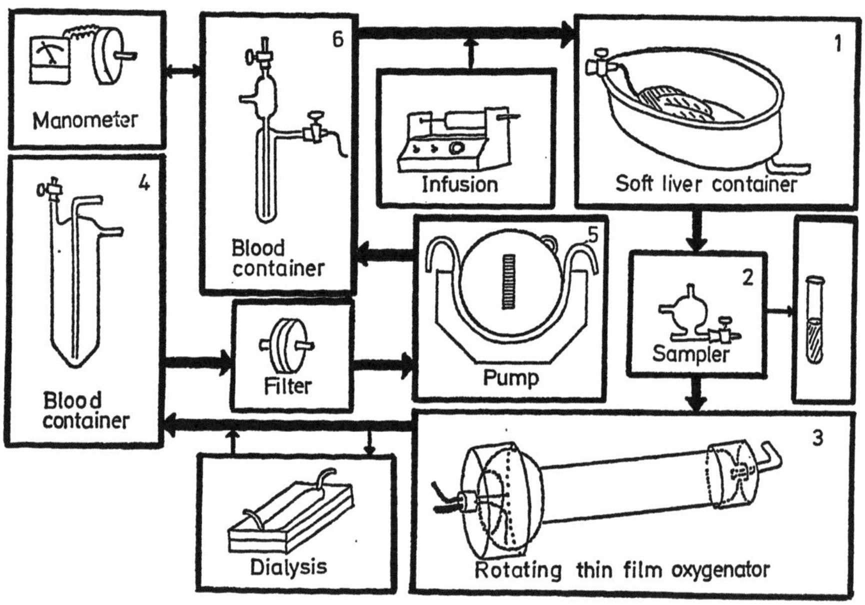

Fig. 1. Functional scheme of the perfusion apparatus. The arrows indicate the flow of perfusion medium

The level of the pentobarbital added to the medium decreased by a first-order rate from 10—180 min of liver perfusion (BARTOŠEK *et al.*, 1972 b).

The half-life of pentobarbital (T ½) was 10 times higher when livers isolated from tumor-bearing rats were perfused with blood from the same group of animals than in control experiments with normal rats (Table 1). It was evident from cross experiments (liver obtained from control animals and blood obtained from tumor-bearing animals and *vice versa*) that the metabolic capacity of the liver was also impaired when the blood of tumor-bearing animals was utilized.

A similar situation is revealed by measuring the formation of cyclophosphamide metabolites by the perfused liver. The total quantity of reactive products was measured in terms of nor-HN_2 equivalents (FRIEDMAN and BOGER, 1961) and expressed by the rate constant of their increase in the medium. The presence of Walker carcinosarcoma inhibited the formation of reactive metabolites in the liver. The "inhibitory signal" was also present in blood of tumor-bearing animals as was demonstrated by cross experiments (Table 2). These data were in good agreement with the results obtained *in vivo* (Table 3).

Table 1. Pentobarbital elimination from the medium during rat liver perfusion

Liver	Blood	Half-life of pentobarbital [a] T ½ min
Normal	Normal	32.2 [b]
Walker [c]	Walker	323.0
Normal	Walker	88.0
Walker	Normal	116.5

[a] Initial concentration of pentobarbital was 25 μg/ml of the medium.
[b] Mean of 5 experiments. $p < 0.01$.
[c] Walker 256 carcinosarcoma.

Table 2. Cyclophosphamide transformation during rat liver perfusion [a]

Liver	Blood	First-order rate constant $K_1 \times 10^{-3}\ min^{-1}$
Normal	Normal	30.4 ± 3.5 [b]
Walker [c]	Walker	12.6 ± 0.9
Normal	Walker	18.2 ± 1.3
Walker	Normal	11.4 ± 0.8

[a] Formation of metabolic products expressed in nor-HN_2 equivalents.
[b] Mean of 5 experiments.
[c] Walker 256 carcinosarcoma.
The initial concentration of cyclophosphamide was 150 μg/ml of medium.

Table 3. Concentration of Cyclophosphamide metabolites in rat serum [a]

Min after treatment	mμ moles of nor-HN_2 equivalents/ml	
	Controls	Walker
1	32.0 ± 4.3	47.6 ± 10.0
5	73.9 ± 5.1	47.6 ± 7.8 [b]
10	97.0 ± 4.3	62.5 ± 2.2 [c]
15	103.5 ± 2.8	73.1 ± 3.3 [c]
20	131.5 ± 12.4	78.1 ± 7.8 [b]
40	119.9 ± 2.2	82.2 ± 13.1 [b]
60	93.7 ± 12.4	60.8 ± 7.1
120	18.9 ± 1.6	22.2 ± 2.5
180	<10	12.3 ± 3.8

[a] The drug was administered intravenously in a dose of 80 mg/kg body wt.
[b] $p < 0.05$ with respect to controls.
[c] $p < 0.01$ with respect to controls.

These examples show that in the presence of tumors the rate of metabolism in the liver may be decreased for certain drugs. Nevertheless, the opposite case was also found. The disappearance of hydrocortisone from plasma of rats bearing Walker 256 carcinosarcoma was accelerated *in vivo* in respect to normal rats (MARC *et al.*, (1973). Accordingly the metabolic capacity of livers obtained from tumor-bearing rats was found to be increased for this drug.

This was more evident with 9000 xg liver fraction of tumor bearing rats (78.5 ± 3.6% clearance) than in analogous control experiments with normal animals (52.6 ± 3.4% clearance).

Increased elimination of hydrocortisone from the medium was also found during the perfusion of isolated livers, i.e. the half-life (T ½) of this steroid was shorter in tumor-bearing rats than in controls. Cross experiments demonstrated that in this case the blood of tumor bearing animals did not influence the metabolic activity of liver tissue (Table 4).

Table 4. Hydrocortisone elimination from the medium during rat liver perfusion

Liver	Blood	Half-life of hydrocortisone T ½ min
Normal	Normal	22.4 ± 0.4 [b]
Walker [c]	Walker	12.8 ± 1.2
Normal	Walker	23.8 ± 0.1
Walker	Normal	13.5 ± 1.8

[a] Initial concentration of hydrocortisone was 20 µg/ml of medium.
[b] Mean of 5 experiments.
[c] Walker 256 carcinosarcoma.

Table 5. Blood levels of 6-mercaptopurine in rats [a]

Min after treatment	6-mercaptopurine concn. µg/ml	
	Controls	Walker
1	95.1 ± 2.1	41.6 ± 1.4 [b]
5	23.6 ± 1.6	10.1 ± 0.9 [b]
15	15.9 ± 2.6	1.2 ± 0.5 [b]
30	3.3 ± 0.7	0.5 ± 0.3

[a] The drug was administered intravenously in a dose of 80 mg/kg body wt.
[b] $p < 0.01$ relative to controls. Each figure represents an average of 5 assays.

Some discrepancies between the *in vivo* and the *in vitro* results should also be mentioned. We expected in view of the results obtained *in vivo* (Table 5) (DONELLI *et al.*, 1972) that the elimination of 6-mercaptopurine would be increased in the perfusion of the liver obtained from tumor-bearing in respect to normal rats. However, no difference could be observed (Table 6).

Table 6. 6-mercaptopurine disappearance from the perfusion medium [a]

Liver	Blood	Half-life of 6-mercaptopurine $T\frac{1}{2}$ min
Normal	Normal	42.5 ± 5.6 [b]
Walker	Walker	34.6 ± 3.6

[a] Initial concentration of 6-mercaptopurine was 50 μg/ml of perfusion medium.
[b] Mean of 6 experiments. $p < 0.05$.

It is very difficult to explain these various findings in a simple manner. The decreased metabolism of pentobarbital and of cyclophosphamide may be consequent upon the release of an "inhibitory signal" from the growing tumor that decreases the activity of liver microsomal enzymes, perhaps by affecting the synthesis or the activity of one or more of the components necessary for the electron transport chain mediated by cytochrome P_{450}.

On the other hand the presence of the tumor may be regarded as a continuous stress which increases the production of corticosteroids. The enhanced levels of these hormones may elicit "autoinduction" of the enzymes which metabolize them in the liver (MARC *et al.*, 1973).

The metabolism of pyrimidines and purines is under a strict cellular control that limits their uptake to the necessary amounts. The effect observed *in vivo* may therefore take place in tissues other than the liver (DONELLI *et al.*, 1972).

This altered metabolism in the liver due to the presence of a tumor may be enhanced by extrahepatic mechanisms that contribute to the debilitation of the tumor host. An example of this situation may be the increased mobilization of free fatty acids which depletes the triglycerides stored in the adipose tissue of rats bearing Walker carcinosarcoma (BIZZI *et al.*, 1968).

It is beyond the scope of this presentation to describe and to analyze all the changes induced in the host by the presence of a tumor.

On the basis of the experimental data presented here, the following conclusions may be drawn:

1. The capacity of the liver to metabolize different compounds both *in vivo* and *in vitro* is changed in tumor-bearing animals relative to normal animals.

2. The rate of drug metabolism in the liver may either increase (e.g. hydrocortisone, 6-mercaptopurine) or decrease (e.g. pentobarbital, cyclophosphamide) in the presence of a tumor.

3. Use of the technique of isolated liver perfusion in determining the observed changes of drug disposition makes it possible to establish separately for blood and liver the extent of participation.

Acknowledgement

The work here described has been supported by NIH Contract No. NCI-C-723242 and by Contract No. 71.00821.04 of the Consiglio Nazionale delle Ricerche.

References

Bartošek, I., Guaitani, A., Garattini, S.: Long-term perfusion of isolated rat liver. Pharmacology **8**, 244 (1972 a).

Bartošek, I., Guaitani, A., Donelli, M. G.: Prolonged metabolism of pentobarbital in isolated perfused liver of tumor-bearing rats. Biochem. Pharmacol. **21**, 2359 (1972 b).

Bartošek, I., Marc, V., Guaitani, A., Garattini, S.: Accelerated catabolism of hydrocortisone in isolated perfused liver of tumor-bearing rats. Biochem. Pharmacol. **22**, 2429 (1973).

Bizzi, A., Garattini, S., Guaitani, A.: Mobilization of plasma free fatty acids during the growth of various experimental tumors. Europ. J. Cancer **4**, 117 (1968).

Donelli, M. G., Colombo, T., Forgione, A., Garattini, S.: Distribution of 6-mercaptopurine in tumor-bearing animals. Pharmacology **8**, 311 (1972).

Friedman, O. M., Boger, E.: Colorimetric estimation of nitrogen mustards in aqueous media. Hydrolytic behaviour of bis/beta-chlorethyl/amine, nor-HN2. Anal. Chem. **33**, 906 (1961).

Marc, V., Donelli, M. G., Bartošek, I., Guaitani, A., Morselli, P. L.: Metabolism of exogenous cortisol in tumor-bearing rats. Europ. J. Cancer (in press).

Rosso, R., Dolfini, E., Donelli, M. G.: Prolonged effect of pentobarbital in tumor-bearing rats. Europ. J. Cancer **4**, 133 (1968).

Rosso, R., Donelli, M. G., Franchi, G., Garattini, S.: Impairment of drug metabolism in tumor-bearing animals. Europ. J. Cancer **7**, 565 (1971).

Is Local Chemotherapy Less Toxic than Systemic?

P. J. SINDRAM

Centre National de la Recherche Scientifique (C.N.R.S.), Paris/France

In recent years the superiority of intra-arterial administration of cytotoxic drugs over their systemic use has been questioned. Clinical evaluation has not been possible because of the small number of patients treated in each separate center and the lack of standardization of drug schedules. It therefore seemed important to get further information from animal experiment's. The following questions were asked:

1. It is possible to set up an animal model suitable for continuous intra-arterial infusion with methotrexate (MTX)?

2. In this model, is the anti-tumor effect of regional continuous intra-arterial infusion of MTX superior to continuous systemic administration.

In the rat, occlusive catheterization of a common carotid artery provides a good model for regional infusion of a rhabdomyosarcoma transplanted in one auricle. A

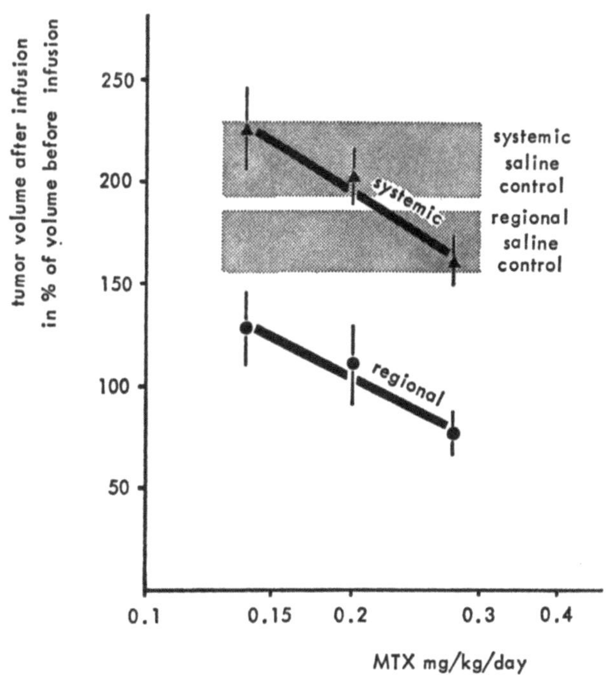

Fig. 1. Intra arterial treatment with MTX

symmetrically transplanted tumor in the other auricle makes it possible to measure the anti-tumor effects of systemic MTX in the same animal. The catheter is implanted in such a way that the rat cannot pull it out and yet can move freely within its cage.

The results are presented for continuous infusion of MTX for 7 days at 3 dose levels; the doses are plotted horizontally on a logarithmic scale (Fig. 1) and mortality (not noted in the figure) is about 0%, 50% and 100%, respectively. Tumor volume after 7 days infusion is indicated on the ordinate as percentage of tumor volume at the beginning of an infusion. The shaded areas indicate the increase in tumor volume during 7 days of saline control infusion. At all dose levels on the local infusion side, we see significantly less increase in tumor volume over the value for the saline control. On the systemic side only the highest dose gives significantly less increase in volume compared with the saline control infusion.

If we extrapolate backward the line that represents the effect of local infusion of MTX, we get on that line the same effects as with systemic MTX at a 2.89 times lower dose. However, part of this effect is also seen with saline. If we apply a correction for this saline effect, the real gain with intra-arterial infusion in this model is a factor of 2.0.

Further studies are planned to evaluate MTX in combination with Leucovorin.

Acknowledgement

These studies were initiated at the Radiobiological Institute at Rijswijk (Holland) with a grant from the "Konigin Wilhelmina Fonds", and continued at the Laboratory of Experimental Medicine, Free University of Amsterdam (Holland).

Pharmacokinetic Simulation: A Future Means for Better Control of Cancer Chemotherapy*

TH. LINCOLN and E. J. FREIREICH

University of Texas, M.D. Anderson Hospital and Tumor Institut, Houston, TX

In chemotherapy we should like to have a methodology which is the analogy to modern radiation dosimetry. In radiation therapy we calculate not only how much radiation comes out of the x-ray port but how much reaches each tissue of interest. In chemotherapy we would like to know not only the dose per square meter of the drug we have introduced into the patient but also how the drug is distributed. What is the concentration as a function of time in the tumor and in tissues which are susceptible to side effects? What is the effect of tissue metabolism on the blood concentration and on the drug distribution? Pharmacokinetics, and pharmacokinetics simulation by computer, promises to provide such a tool.

In 1968 DEDRICK and BISCHOFF (1968) correctly observed that the dominant feature determining the distribution of drugs by the blood stream is the rate of blood flow to a tissue as compared with the volume of that tissue. The distribution may be further modified by protein or tissue binding characteristics of the drug which can change the rate of diffusion. In the simplest cases, however, diffusion effects are rapid as compared to the effects of blood flow and thus the presence of secondary binding does not effect distribution. The concentration in a tissue is also effected by the metabolism in that tissue which in turn effects the concentration in the blood. It is possible to set up a system of differential equations which describe the changes in concentration of drugs as a function of time in the blood and in each tissue. These equations have the following form:

$$\frac{dCT}{dt} \cdot VT = QBT.\,CB - QBT.\,CT - \text{Metabolism} + KT$$

where CT is the concentration in the tissue, VT is the total volume of the tissue and the venous blood in equilibrium with it, QBT is the rate of blood flow to the tissue, CB the concentration in the blood, and CT the concentration in the tissue. KT is a term which describes the special characteristics of a particular tissue, such as urinary clearance in the kidney or biliary excretion in the liver. The metabolic term is defined as a Michaelis-Menten equation of the following form:

$$\text{Metabolism} = VMAXT \cdot VTA \cdot CT/KMT + CT)$$

* This work is supported by NIH Grant No. CA-12369.

where VMAXT is the maximum metabolic rate, VTA the volume of the tissue which is metabolically active (usually the tissue minus the blood), and KMT is the Michaelis constant.

Clearly, if every tissue is a compartment, these models have very many parameters, but the advantage is that these parameters can be obtained from *in vivo* and *in vitro* experiments in man, or by a physiological scaling of data obtained on animals. In this manner the distribution of thiopental following injection of a known dose has been accurately modeled (BISCHOFF and DEDRICK, 1968), as has the distribution of a much more complicated drug, methotrexate (BISCHOFF and DEDRICK, 1971).

Our contribution has been to provide an interactive computer modeling system using computer graphics to carry out such simulations and to explore the various

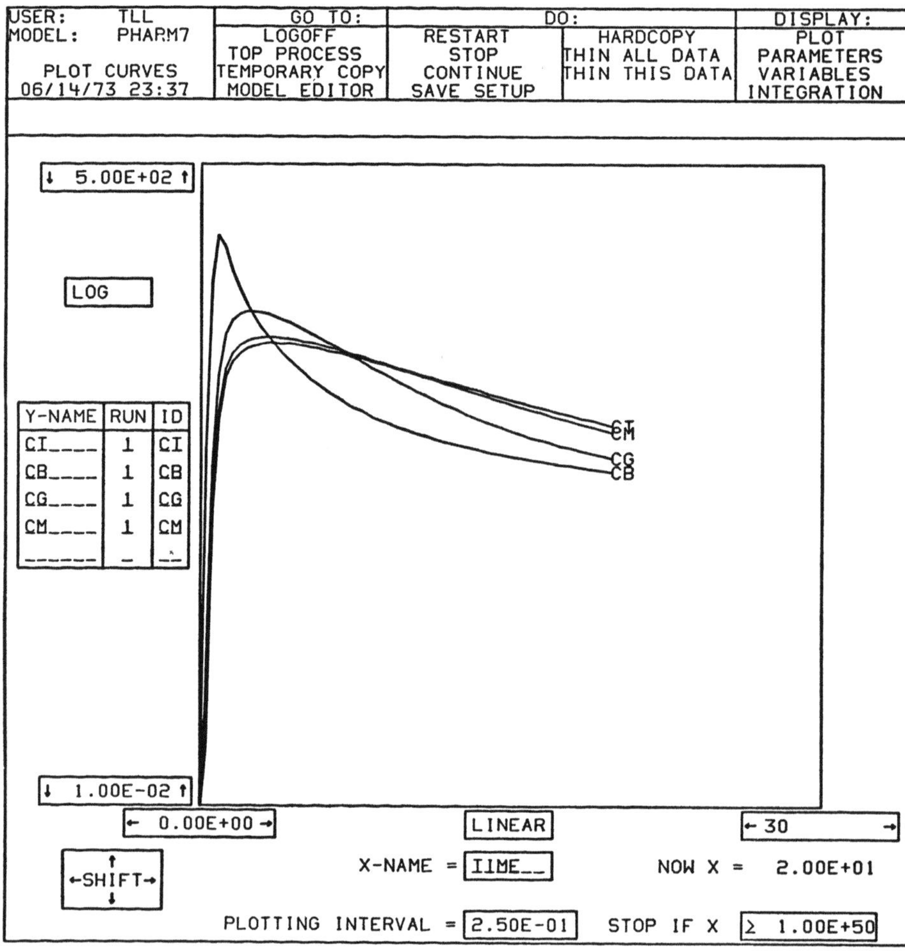

Fig. 1. BIOMOD graphics display of cytosine arabinoside pharmacokinetic simulation in 70 kg man. Dose: 100 mg/meter². Ordinate: Concentration of drug on logarithmic scale. Abscissa: Time in minutes. CT = Concentration in testicular tissues; CB = Blood; CG = Gut; CM = Bone marrow. Note similarity of testis to marrow

ramifications of such models (LINCOLN *et al.*, 1973). For this we have used a RAND-developed biological modeling system called BIOMOD (GRONER and CLARK, 1971). This is a very general computer graphics modeling package which allows the construction of models in an organized modular way using flow diagrams, and offers a means of programming in mathematical equations rather than, for example, in FORTRAN. Pharmacokinetics is but a single example of its capacities.

We present here simulation results which show the concentration of cytosine arabinoside as a function of time in various body compartments in a 70 kg man. It extends some work previously reported by LINCOLN *et al.* At a recent meeting Professor Mathé asked me to examine a testis compartment, to study the concentration *vs.* time curves for that organ, and to consider ways of improving the effectiveness of drug impact on the testicular tissue.

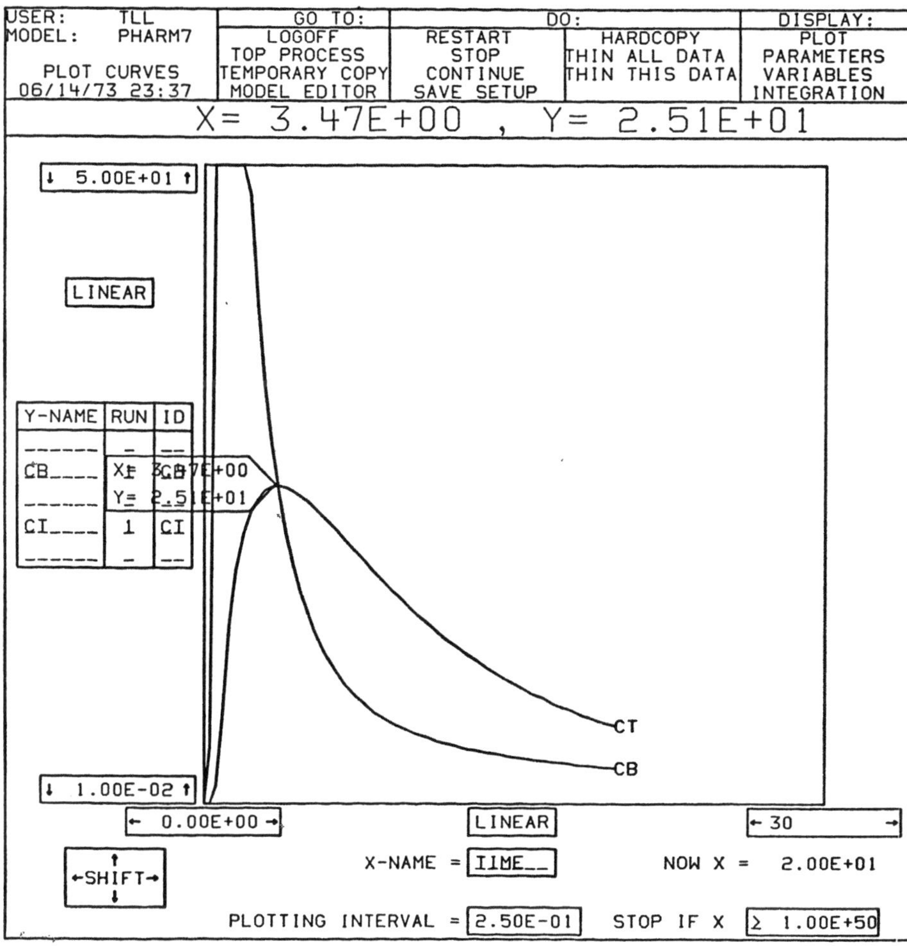

Fig. 2. BIOMOD display with linear scale of drug concentration. Pointer identifies maximum concentration in testis at ~ 3.5 min after start of simulated 1 min injection of cytosine arabinoside

If the suggestion is indeed correct, then the results of these computations are particularly satisfying: a rather complicated and expensive analysis leads to a simple clinical rule of thumb which is low in cost and easy to perform.

We extended our previous model by creating the appropriate differential equation for the testis and introducing the best values available to us for the parameters. To modify the model took less than thirty minutes at the computer console. The major effort required was to find good data on the testis. Professor EIK-NES at USC was able to provide us with the most accurate information. The blood flow rate in mammals appears to be a constant of 1.5 ml of blood per 10 g of tissue per minute (EIK-NES, comm.). Organ sizes were taken from MAPLESON (1963). In the absence of data on the metabolism of cytosine arabinoside by the testis, it was considered to be negligible, although this may not be the case.

The simulation predicts the concentration *vs.* time to be almost the same as that predicted for the bone-marrow, given assumptions of normal physiology (Fig. 1). The testis, however, offers two fortuitous advantages because it is an external and isolated organ. First, it should be possible to validate the hypothetical simulated results by cannulating the superficial testicular vein and observing the changes in concentration of the drug directly. Given the model, this blood would be presumed to be in equilibrium with the testis. Further, the nature of the model suggests a means of altering the exposure of the tissue to the drug. It will be noted from Fig. 1 that the peak concentration of the drug corresponds to the point where the concentration in the blood falls below the concentration in the tissue. In qualitative terms, the circulation of the blood through the tissue increases the concentration in the tissue so long as the concentration in the blood is higher, and diminishes the tissue concentration later when the concentration in the blood is lower. Thus it should be possible to maintain the concentration in the tissue at the maximum level (or at least to reduce its fall, if metabolism occurs) if the circulation is cut off for an acceptable period of time just as the maximum concentration is reached. In this case, pharmacokinetic simulation leads to a concrete medical suggestion: increased drug exposure should be achieved by manually occluding the circulation to the testis at the base of the scrotum approximately 3.5 min after the start of a 1-min intravenous injection of cytosine arabinoside. The time of 3.5 min is the maximum obtained from a simulation which includes, in addition to the differential equations for distribution, an injection function to simulate the i.v. push (BELLMAN *et al.*, 1960), a Laplace transform to simulate initial blood mixing based on dye dilution experiments (ZIERLER, 1962), and an 8-sec delay for the venous transfer from the antecubital fossa (see Fig. 2).

References

BELLMAN, R., JAQUEZ, J., KALABA, R.: Some mathematical aspects of chemotherapy: I. One-organ models. Bull. Mathematical Biophysics. **22**, 181 (1960).

BISCHOFF, K., DEDRICK, R., ZAHARKO, D., LONGSTRETH, J.: Methotrexate pharmacokinetics. J. pharm. Sci. 60, 8, 1128 (1971).

BISCHOFF, K., DEDRICK, R.: Thiopental pharmacokinetics. J. pharm. Sci. **57**, 8, 1346 (1968).

DEDRICK, R., BISCHOFF, K.: Pharmacokinetics in application of the artificial kidney. Chem. Eng. Prog. Symp. **84**, 64, 32 (1968).

GRONER, G., CLARK, R.: BIOMOD: An interactive graphics system for analysis through simulation.pp, 197—201. Miami Beach, Florida: Proceedings of the 1971 IEEE Conf. on Decision and Control.

LINCOLN, T., HARRIS, P., GROSS, J. F.: BIOMOD simulation of pharmacokinetics for leukemia chemotherapy. P-4969. The RAND Corp., 1973.

MAPLESON, W.: An electric analogue for uptake and exchange of inert gases and other agents. J. appl. Physiol. **18**, 197 (1963).

ZIERLER, KENNETH, L.: Circulation times and the theory of indicator dilution methods for determining blood flow and volume. In: Handbook of Physiology, Sec. 2: Circulation Vol. I, pp. 585—615. Washington, D. C.: American Physiological Society 1962.

Carcinogenesis by Cancer Chemotherapeutic Agents: Second Malignancies Complicating Hodgkin's Disease in Remission

G. P. CANELLOS, V. T. DEVITA, J. C. ARSENEAU, and R. C. JOHNSON

Medicine, Radiation Branches, National Cancer Institute, Bethesda, MD

Introduction

It has been long known that in some types of malignant disease there exists an associated propensity to develop other malignant tumors. Acute leukemia complicating the course of polycythemia vera and the increased incidence of skin cancer in chronic lymphocytic leukemia are well known (MODAN, 1965; HYMAN, 1969). It has remained enigmatic whether the disease renders the host more likely to develop second tumors or whether the therapy itself in certain settings, is capable of inducing genetic changes which subsequently lead to malignant degeneration. The importance of second tumor induction emerges only if the patient with advanced disease can survive, with treatment, long enough to increase his risk. This is especially true in the atomic bomb radiation induced leukemias where a latent period of over 5 years was required before an increased incidence of leukemia was noted (BIZZOZERO *et al.*, 1966).

In the last ten years, advances in the treatment of Hodgkin's disease have involved the intensive application of radiation or chemotherapy in high dosage and over long periods of time (KAPLAN *et al.*, 1966). The resultant prolonged disease-free survival of patients with both advanced and localized disease have made available a study population which have received these intensive modalities alone or in combination and thus permit an assessment of the incidence of new malignancies in these populations.

Methods

Four hundred and thirty eight cases of Hodgkin's disease treated and followed at NCI were divided into subgroups according to the type of treatment received and the incidence of new second malignancies recorded. The data are calculated on the basis of age, sex and man-years of observation and the expected risk of developing second tumors derived from the Third National Cancer Survey of 1969. The data are expressed as ratios of the observed over the expected incidence. The

2 patients who developed acute myeloid leukemia had cytogenic studies performed by Dr. J. WHANG-PENG, 1970, NCI.

The category of intensive chemotherapy (IC) includes patients who received at least 6 monthly cycles of combination chemotherapy (MOPP) according to dosage schedules previously reported (DEVITA *et al.*, 1970).

Intensive radiation therapy includes the application of at least 3000 r in a unified course of treatment to all axial lymph node regions (total nodal irradiation); primary involved nodes plus contiguous nodes area (extended field irradiation). The group which received both IR + IC was comprised of basically two types: 1. Patients who presented with localized disease, received intensive radiotherapy, subsequently relapsed with systemic disease and thus treated with intensive chemotherapy (IC and 2. patients with IIIB Hodgkin's disease who were treated on a protocol which included at least 6 months cycles of MOPP to complete remission and, after a 3—7 month rest period in remission, treated with total nodal irradiation (CANELLOS *et al.*, 1972). Abbreviations are listed in Fig. 1.

IC = Intensive Chemotherapy Cyclic Combination – MOPP

IR = Intensive Radiotherapy (>3500r)

*** { Mantle / Mantle Plus Extended Field / Total Nodal**

***Given as a Unified Course**

Fig. 1. Abbreviations for different treatments

Results

A total of 14 second tumors were noted in 438 patients after the initiation of therapy. The distribution of numbers of tumors according to the type of treatment and duration of follow-up in man-years of observation is shown in Fig. 2. The data are compared to the expected incidence. It can be seen that patients who received both intensive radiation therapy and intensive chemotherapy (IR + IC) had a 10.4% second cancer incidence compared to 2.3% in the remaining sub-groups. The data assume greater significance when analyzed according to the expected incidence for the age groups at risk and the observation period. At this point in time, patients in the sub-group IR + IC have 23 times higher incidence of tumors over the expected. These numbers are quite significant ($p < 0.05$). Fig. 3 divides the composition of this high risk group according to the intervening duration between the administration of the intensive therapies. The majority of cases occurred in the group where relapse of Hodgkin's disease occurred between therapies (IR → IC). This may have some significance if one assumes that a degree of Hodgkin's disease-related impaired cellular immunity can contribute to the oncogenic factors. The types of tumors seen are listed in Fig. 4. All were highly malignant and fatal including two cases of acute myeloid leukemia.

The cytogenetic studies of both leukemic patients are outlined in the Table. It is of note that both patients demonstrated grossly similar aneuploid cell lines of

HODGKIN'S DISEASE

RISK OF SECOND MALIGNANCY WITH INTENSIVE THERAPY

Major Mode(s) of Therapy	Number of Patients	Observation Period (man years)	Number of Second Tumors OBS	EXP	OBS/EXP
IR	149	562	4	1.05	3.8*
IC	110	371	3	0.94	3.2
IR + IC	48	171	5	0.21	23.0*
NIT	131	543	2	1.28	1.6

IR = Total nodal or extended field radiotherapy — *$P < 0.05$

IC = MOPP or COPP chemotherapy for a minimum of 6 months

NIT = No intensive therapy

Fig. 2. The risk of second malignancies according to treatment groups

HODGKIN'S DISEASE
SECOND TUMORS

Sequence of Treatment	Total Patients	Mean Interval (Months)	Second Malignancy
IR → IC	26	22	4
IC → IR	22	7	1

Fig. 3. Second tumors in Hodgkin's receiving both intensive therapies in different sequences

HODGKIN'S DISEASE

SECOND MALIGNANCIES AFTER INTENSIVE RADIOTHERAPY AND CHEMOTHERAPY

Case	Time from completion of therapy to diagnosis of second malignancy (months)			Histologic Diagnosis
	Radiotherapy	→	MOPP	
W.W. 53/m	17		9	Squamous cell carcinoma–Skin
J.McC. 23/m	5		4	Undifferentiated mucin-secreting carcinoma–Lung
E.B. 18/m	3		2	Fibrosarcoma–Chest wall
L.W. 19/f	17	←	28	Acute Myelomonocytic Leukemia
R.H. 27/m	36		7	Acute Myeloblastic Leukemia

Fig. 4. Various types of cancer complicating the course of Hodgkin's disease

Table. Cytogenetics of acute myeloid leukemia complicating Hodgkin's disease

	Chromosome number		
R. H. 27 M	44	45	46
12/26/72	2	7 (C-)	13
1/30/73		3 (C-1)	1
L. D. 21 F			
2/6/73		45	46
		38 (C-)	2
3/13/73		5 (C-)	

(C-) = Missing chromosome in C group.

45 chromosomes with a missing chromosome in the C group. Chromosome banding studies were not performed so that it is not possible to determine whether the defects were identical in both patients.

Discussion

The potential for an increased risk of developing second malignancies in the course of Hodgkin's disease has been considered in the past (RAZIS *et al.*, 1959; MOERTEL and HAGEDORN, 1957; BERG, 1967). The overall incidence ranges from 1.6—2.2% in reported series. These analyses failed to define the role of therapy as a possible factor in tumor induction. A previous report from our group defined a highly significant difference between the incidence of second tumors in patients who received both intensive radiation and chemotherapy. In that report no cases of acute leukemia were noted (ARSENEAU *et al.*, 1972). Since then we have expanded our IR+IC group from 35 to 48 patients at risk and have noted two cases of acute leukemia. Despite an expanded man-years of observation the highly significant correlation is maintained.

Our observations indicate that patients with Hodgkin's disease do indeed have a higher incidence of second tumors than the general population and further, that one treatment subgroup has a considerably higher risk than all the others.

It is difficult to precisely define an oncogenic mechanism in these patients since at least three factors may be involved. First, there is the known impairment of cellular immunity which characterizes advanced Hodgkin's disease (YOUNG *et al.*, 1972). Certain congenital diseases with immunologic deficiency as well as chronic lymphocytic leukemia appear to have an increased risk of second tumor (GATTI and GOOD, 1971). Second, the immunosuppressive effects of radiation and chemotherapy are well known (BORELLA *et al.*, 1971). The MOPP regimen entails 2 weekly rest periods off treatment during a monthly course which may permit some repair of immunosuppression or rebound of immunocompetence. There is known to be increased incidence of cerebral histiocytic lymphoma in renal transplant patients where chronic, continuous immunosuppression is applied (DOAK *et al.*, 1968). Perhaps it is significant that a greater number of tumors occurred in patients who experienced an intervening relapse of their disease between intensive therapies. Third, there is the direct cellular affects of these treatments on genetic structures of the cell. The increased incidence of leukemia following radiation from the atomic explosions in Japan, and following therapeutic application for ankylosing spondylitis is well defined (COURT-BROWN and DOLL, 1957). Cancer chemotherapy in man has not been clearly associated with second cancers perhaps because these are drugs that are usually administered to patients with advanced malignancy and limited prognosis. However, long term follow-up of women cured of gestational neoplasms with methotrexate therapy has not shown an increase risk on second cancer (ROSS and LIPSETT). Recently the occurrence of acute leukemia in the course of multiple myeloma has suggested that perhaps chronic oral alkylating agents treatment may be an oncogenic factor (KYLE *et al.*, 1970). Further the drug procarbazine which is included in the MOPP regimen has a marked carcinogenic effect in experimental animals (O'GARA *et al.*, 1971). This agent is also immunosuppressive.

It should be noted that the five second tumors in our IR+IC series all occurred in the regions where intensive radiation was applied including the bone marrow. Cytogenetic studies revealed consistent chromosomal defects in both leukemic patients which, in part, could be direct effects of these treatments. In general, the chromosomal aberrations associated with radiation are random and nonspecific (WARREN and MEISNER, 1965). The C group (6-X-12) is the largest single subgroup of chromosomes and thus might be more likely to be modified by ionizing radiation and drugs. However, in two large series of cytogenetic studies in acute myeloid leukemia, 45 (C-) chromosome leukemic cell lines occurred in 8 out of 198 patients studied (WHANG-PENG *et al.*, 1970; HART *et al.*, 1971). Aneuploidy itself is not uncommon, occurring in about $^1/_3$ of all patients. The C group has also been noted to yield significant abnormalities such as monosomy and trisomy in patients with preleukemia and children with myeloproliferative disorders (ROWLEY *et al.*, 1966; HOLDEN *et al.*, 1971; TEASDALE *et al.*, 1970; JACKSON *et al.*, 1967; SANDBERG *et al.*, 1964; WINKELSTEIN *et al.*, 1966).

A few cases of acute myeloid leukemia have been reported to complicate the course of Hodgkin's disease. The Mayo clinic group found four cases of acute myelomonocytic leukemia in 1500 cases of Hodgkin's disease occurring $1^1/_2$, 4, $5^1/_2$, and 18 years after the primary diagnosis (NEWMAN *et al.*, 1970). This latter series, if the follow-up is complete, represents the only other published series from which the occurrence rate can be estimated. Chromosome studies performed in one patient with acute myeloid leukemia, who had previously received radiation therapy and nitrogen mustard, failed to reveal an aneuploid cell line (EZDINLI *et al.*, 1969).

In conclusion, the results suggest that intensive treatment with radiation and cytotoxic drugs may render patients with Hodgkin's disease more likely to develop second malignancies. These observations would not be possible unless these treatments were successful in allowing patients to survive for prolonged periods free to Hodgkin's disease. The grave prognosis of unchecked advanced Hodgkin's disease represents a far greater threat to the patient than the small but statistically increased risk of developing another tumor at some time in the future following successful treatment of the basic disease.

Acknowledgements

The authors wish to express their gratitute to Dr. Jacqueline Whang-Peng for the cytogenetic studies and Doctors R. Sponzo and L. Schnipper for their participation in the initial phase of this study.

References

ARSENEAU, J. C., SPONZO, R. W., LEVIN, D. L., SCHNIPPER, L. E., BONNER, H., YOUNG, R. C., CANELLOS, G. P., JOHNSON, R. E., DEVITA, V. T.: Nonlymphomatous malignant tumors complicating Hodgkin's disease. New Engl. J. Med. **287**, 1119 (1972).

BERG, J. W.: The incidence of multiple primary cancers. I. The development of further cancers in patients with lymphomas, leukemias and myeloma. J. nat. Cancer Inst. **38**, 741 (1967).

BIZZOZERO, O. J., JR., JOHNSON, K. G., CIOCCO, A.: Radiation-related leukemia in Hiroshima and Nagasaki, 1946—1964. New Engl. J. Med. **274**, 1095 (1966).

BORELLA, L., WEBSTER, R. G.: The immunosuppressive effects of long-term combination chemotherapy in children with acute leukemia in remission. Cancer Res. **31**, 420 (1971).

CANELLOS, G. P., YOUNG, R. C., DEVITA, V. T.: Combination chemotherapy for advanced Hodgkin's disease in relapse following extensive radiotherapy. Clin. Pharm. Therap. **13**, 750 (1972).

COURT-BROWN, W. M., DOLL, R.: Leukemia and aplastic anemia in patients irradiated for ankylosing spondylitis. Med. Res. Counc. Spec. Rep. **295**, 1 (1957).

DEVITA, V. T., SERPICK, A. A., CARBONE, P. P.: Combination chemotherapy in the treatment of advanced Hodgkin's disease. Ann. intern. Med. **73**, 881 (1970).

DOAK, P. B., MONTGOMERIE, J. Z., NORTH, J. D. K., SMITH, F.: Reticulum cell sarcoma after renal homotransplantation and azathioprine and prednisone therapy. Brit. med. J. **1968 IV**, 746.

EZDINLI, E. Z., SOKAL, J. E., AUNGST, C. W., KIM, U., DANBERG, A. A.: Myeloid leukemia in Hodgkin's disease: Chromosomal abnormalities. Ann. intern. Med. **71**, 1097 (1969).

GATTI, R. A., GOOD, R. A.: Occurrence of malignancy in immunodeficiency diseases. Cancer **1**, 89 (1971).

HART, J. S., TRUJILLO, J. M., FREIREICH, E. J., GEORGE, S. L., FREI, E.: Cytogenetic studies and their clinical correlates in adults with acute leukemia. Ann. intern. Med. **75**, 353 (1971).

HOLDEN, J. D., GARCIA, F. U., SAMUELS, M., DUPIN, C., STALLWORTH, B., ANDERSON, E.: Myelofibrosis with C. monosomy of marrow elements in a child. Amer. J. clin. Path. **55**, 573 (1971).

HYMAN, G. A.: Increased incidence of neoplasia in association with chronic lymphocytic leukemia. Scand. J. Haemat. **6**, 99 (1969).

JACKSON, J. F., HIGGINS, L.: Group C. monosomy in myelofibrosis with myeloid metaplasia. Arch. intern. Med. **119**, 403 (1967).

KAPLAN, H. S.: Role of intensive radiotherapy in the management of Hodgkin's disease. Cancer (Philad.) **19**, 356 (1966).

KYLE, R. A., PIERRE, R. V., BAYRD, E. D.: Multiple myeloma and acute myelomonocytic leukemia; report of four cases possibly related to melphalan. New. Engl. J. Med. **21**, 1121 (1970).

LACHER, M. J., SUSSMAN, L. N.: Leukemia and Hodgkin's disease. Ann. intern. Med. **59**, 369 (1963).

MODAN, B.: Radiophosphorus therapy in polycythemia vera. Blood **26**, 383 (1965).

MOERTEL, C. G., HAGEDORN, A. B.: Leukemia or lymphoma and coexistent primary malignant lesions: a review of the literature and study of 120 cases. Blood **12**, 788 (1957).

NEWMAN, D. R., MALDONADO, J. E., HARRISON, E. G., KIELY, J. M., LINMAN, J. W.: Myelomonocytic leukemia in Hodgkin's disease. Cancer (Philad.) **25**, 128 (1970).

O'GARA, R., ADAMSON, R. H., KELLY, M. G., DALGARD, D. W.: Neoplasms of the hematopoietic system in nonhuman primates: report of one spontaneous tumor and two leukemias induced by procarbazine. J. nat. Cancer Inst. **46**, 1121 (1971).

OSTA, S., WELLS, M., VIAMONTE, M., HARKNESS, D.: Hodgkin's disease termination in acute leukemia. Cancer (Philad.) **26**, 795 (1970).

RAZIS, D. V., DIAMOND, H. D., CRAVER, L. F.: Hodgkin's disease associated with other malignant tumors and certain non-neoplastic diseases. Amer. J. med. Sci. **238**, 327 (1959).

ROSS, G. T., LIPSETT, M.: Personal communications.

ROWLEY, J. D., BLAISDELL, R. K., JACOBSON, L. O.: Chromosome studies in preleukemia I. Aneuploidy of group C. Chromosomes in three patients. Blood **27**, 782 (1966).

SANDBERG, A. A., ISHIHARA, K., CROSSWHITE, L. H.: Group-C trisomy in myeloid metaplasia with possible leukemia. Blood **24**, 716 (1964).

TEASDALE, J. M., WORTH, A. J., COREY, M. J.: A missing group C chromosome in the bone marrow cells of three children with myeloproliferative disease. Cancer (Philad.) **25**, 1468 (1970).

WARREN, S., MEISNER, L.: Chromosomal changes in leukocytes of patients receiving irradiation therapy. J. Amer. med. Ass. **193**, 351 (1965).

WHANG-PENG, J., HENDERSON, E. S., KNUTSEN, T., FREIREICH, E. J., GART, J. J.: Cytogenetic studies in acute myelocytic leukemia with special emphasis on the occurrence of Ph^1 chromosome. Blood **36**, 448, 457 (1970).

WINKELSTEIN, A., SPARKES, R. S., CRADDOCK, C. G.: Trisomy of group C in a myeloproliferative disorder report of case. Blood **27**, 722 (1966).

YOUNG, R. C., CORDER, M. P., HAYNES, H. A., DEVITA, V. T.: Delayed hypersensitivity in Hodgkin's disease. Amer. J. Med. **52**, 63 (1972).

Malignancies Possibly Secondary to Anticancer Therapy

D. Belpomme [1], P. Carde [1], R. K. Oldham [1], G. Mathé [1], C. Jacquillat [2], N. Chelloul [2], M. Weil [2], G. Auclerc [2], C. Weisgerber [2], T. Tanzer [2], and J. Bernard [2]

Institut de Cancérologie et d'Immunogénétique, Hôpital Paul-Brousse, Villejuif [1], and Institut de Recherches sur les Leucemies et les Maladies du Sang, Hôpital Saint-Louis, Paris [2]

The risk of inducing malignancies in man by modern anticancer therapy is becoming an increasingly important problem. It has been known since the beginning of this century that irradiation may be carcinogenic in animals as well as in man (Anderson *et al.*, 1951; Auerbach *et al.*, 1951; Cahan *et al.*, 1948; Court Brown and Doll, 1957; Ghalib *et al.*, 1960; Hempelmann, 1968; Oldham and Polmar, 1973; Swaay, 1965; Totten, 1957) (Table 1). In addiiton, during the last ten years

Table 1. Leukemia and cancers occurring after radiation therapy

Irradiation by external source Tumors	Delay (yr)
— Squamous cell carcinoma	— 5
— Osteosarcoma and other sarcoma	— 15
— Leukemia	— 5—10
— Thyroid adenocarcinoma	— 7—10
— Other carcinomas	— 7—10
Irradiation by internal source	
— Ostéosarcomas by radio therapy	
— Leukemia (?) by ^{131}I or ^{32}P therapy	

there have been a growing number of reports of second malignancies in patients receiving chemotherapeutic agents (Allans, 1970; Catovsky and Galton, 1971; Feingold and Koss, 1969; Garfield, 1970; Smit and Meyler, 1970) (Table 2).

One may argue that the development of second cancers in these patients is related to the patient himself and not to the anticancer therapy (Berg, 1967). However, the recent observation of a very high incidence of malignancy in organ transplant patients receiving chemotherapeutic agents as immunosuppressive therapy deserves attention (Table 3) (Jalota and Eichwald, 1972; McKhann, 1969; Penn, 1970; Simmons and Najarian, 1970; Starzl *et al.*, 1970).

The present report is concerned with the experiences of two anticancer treatment centers (Institut de Cancérologie et d'Immunogénétique [1], Villejuif, and Institut de Recherches sur les Leucemies et les Maladies du Sang, Hôpital Saint Louis [3], Paris). In a retrospective case review we have found 28 cases with dual malignancies over a 12 year period. 10 cases originated at I.C.I.G. and 18 at l'Hôpital Saint Louis.

Table 2. Leukemia or cancers occurring after chemotherapy

Alkylating agents	
β-chloroethylamines	
— p-bis-(chloro-2-ethylamino)-phenyl-butyrique-Ac (Chlorambucil)	— Leukemia
— Cyclophosphamide (Endoxan) (Cytoxan)	— Leukemia
— Melphalan (Alkeran)	— Leukemia
Ethylenes imines	
— Triethylenethiophosphoramide (Thio-Tepa)	— Leukemia
Sulfonic esters	
— Dimethyl-sulfonyloxy 1-4-butane (Myleran-Busulfan)	— Genital cancers (Breast, uterine)
Other drugs	
— Ethylcarbamate (Urethane)	
— Azathioprine (Imuran)	
— MOPP — Procarbazine (Tumorogenic in animal studies	

Table 3. Cancers occurring after immmunosuppressive therapy

Therapeutic agents: Prednisone, Azathioprine, Antilymphocytic Globulins

Tumors:
- — Reticulum cell sarcomas (especially CNS)
- — Superficially located epithelial carcinomas (skin, lip and uterine cervix)
- — Other carcinomas (colon, testis, ovary and stomach)
- — Other sarcomas

Incidence of malignancy:

Tumor	Age (yr)	Ratio of malignancies to No. of:	
		Transplant patients [a]	General population [b]
All malignancies	ALL	650/100,000	139/100,000
Reticulum cell	ALL	400/100,000	0.9/100,000
Sarcoma	Under 40	500/100,000	8.2/100,000

[a] Based on 2000 patient transplants (C. F. MCKHANN).
[b] Connecticut Cancer Registry.

Material and Methods

1. Cases Originated from I.C.I.G.[1]

In the 10 cases, 4 had Hodgkin's disease, 3 breast cancer, 1 carcinoma of the cervix, 1 nephroblastoma (Wilms tumor), and 1 reticulum cell sarcoma, as the primary neoplasia.

7 of these cases developed secondarily acute myeloid leukemia. 2 other patients with Hodgkin's disease developed chronic lymphocytic leukemia and cancer of the breast, whereas the patient with nephroblastoma developed osteosarcoma (Table 4).

Table 4. Secondary neoplasia occurring after treatment

Secondary neoplasia / First neoplasia	Acute leukemia	Chronic leukemia	Breast cancer	Osteo-sarcoma	Total	Chemotherapy and/or radiotherapy	
						Mild	Intensive
Hodgkin's disease	2	1	1		4		4
Breast cancer (Epithelioma and adenocarcinoma)	3				3	1	2
Uterine cervix cancer	1				1	1	
Reticulum cell sarcoma	1				1		1
Wilm's tumor				1	1	1	
Total	7	1	1	1	10	3	7

[a] Experience of Villejuif (G. Mathé).

2. Cases Obtained from Hospital Saint Louis[2]

Among 800 cases with Hodgkin's disease, 18 developed during the follow-up a second cancer or acute leukemia. 6 of these 18 patients presented with acute myeloid leukemia, 2 with Kaposi sarcomas, and 10 a visceral cancer of varying types and localization. In 1 of the patients who developed Kaposi sarcoma, epithelioma of the testis was also discovered simultaneously (Table 5).

3. Diagnostic Criteria

For all patients, the diagnosis of primary and secondary neoplasia was confirmed by examination of biopsy or surgical specimens. Multiple biopsies were examined for the diagnosis of Kaposi sarcoma, and the diagnosis of acute leukemia was established by standard morphological examination of bone marrow aspirations. In addition, bone marrow biopsy was made in 9 cases of acute leukemia.

[1] Director, Professor G. Mathé.
[2] Director, Professor J. Bernard.

Table 5. Secondary tumors occurring after treatment of Hodgkin's disease [a]

Clinical parameters / Secondary disease	No. of patients	Hodgkin's disease: Perceptible phase	Hodgkin's disease: Complete remission	Secondary neoplasia: Death 0	Secondary neoplasia: Death +	Cause of death: Hodgkin	Cause of death: Secondary cancer	Survival after secondary tumor (months)
Leukemia (AML)	6/6		6	1 (?)	5		5	1— 3
Kaposi's sarcoma	2/2	2			2	1	1	5—10
Epithelioma	5/4	1	3	1	3		3	2—36
Adenocarcinoma	6/6	4	2	3	3		3 [b]	1—24
Total	19/18	7	11	5	13	1	12	

[a] Experience of Hôpital St. Louis (J. BERNARD).
[b] One patient died after surgery for secondary tumor.

Table 6. Classification of treatments received by patients according to type and intensity

Intensity of treatment / Type of treatment	Chemotherapy	Radiotherapy
Intensive	More than 2 drugs, with increase of the dose within a period of more than 3 months	Cobalt therapy over more than 2 fields or 200 KV over more than 3 fields
Mild	Less than 2 drugs, with reduction of the dose within less than 3 months	Cobalt therapy over less than 2 fields or 200 KV over less than 3 fields

4. Case Analysis

For each patient the interval (in years) between the first and second malignancies was determined. The precise schedules of different treatments given to each patient were then tabulated. The treatments were arbitrarily classified into four categories according to the type of therapy (chemotherapy, radiotherapy) as well as to the total dose received by the patients (Table 6). In 18 of the cases, radiotherapy was given in combination with chemotherapy. These were separated into groups as follows: Group I: predominantly or solely intensive chemotherapy; Group II: predominantly or solely intensive radiotherapy; Group III: intensive radio and chemotherapy; and Group IV: moderate radio and/or chemotherapy.

Results

1. Leukemia Occurring as a Second Malignancy After Chemo- or Radiation Therapy

Among 28 secondary malignancies, 13 were acute myeloid leukemia. The intervals between malignancies varied from 2 months to 12 years. 3 of the 7 cases from ICIG received intensive radio and chemotherapy. The other four cases received only radiotherapy. This is in contrast to those cases from Hôpital Saint Louis where all 6 patients had received combined chemo and radiotherapy. It is important to note that for all 13 cases, the cytological diagnosis was definitely acute myeloid leukemia and that for 12 of them, the interval between the diagnosis and death was between 1 and 3 months. This poor prognosis appears to be related to the leukemia since all the 6 patients with Hodgkin's disease from Hôpital St. Louis were in complete clinical remission from their Hodgkin's disease at the time the leukemia was discovered (Table 5).

2. Malignancies After Combined Chemo- and Radiotherapy

12 patients with Hodgkin's disease from Hôpital St. Louis developed second malignancies: 6 adenocarcinomas, 5 epitheliomas, and 2 Kaposi sarcomas. The organ involvement and type of second tumor are presented in Table 7. At the time of diagnosis of the second tumor 12 patients were in complete clinical remission from their Hodgkin's disease. Subsequently 8 have died, and for 7 of them, this was due to the second cancer, emphasizing that the prognosis is poor once the diagnosis of the second tumor is established.

3. Relationship Between the Intensity of Treatment and Occurrence of Second Malignancies

7 of the 10 ICIG cases and 15 of the 18 Hôpital St. Louis cases occurred after intensive treatment with either chemotherapy, radiotherapy or both (Table 1, 4 and 8). This suggests that the intensity of therapy may play a role in the development of secondary cancers.

4. The Interval Between the Two Malignancies

Except for 2 cases where the second cancer occurred two months and 31 years after the first, the intervals ranged from 6 months to 12 years. As shown in Table 6, there is no significant difference in the mean delay of second neoplasia occurrence for the 3 types of second malignancies: leukemia, epithelioma or adenocarcinoma. However, there does seem to be a correlation between combined intensive therapy and the early occurrence of the second malignancy. Those receiving both had a mean appearance time of 3.75 years, whereas for those receiving only intensive radiotherapy it was 8.5 years (Table 9).

Table 7. Type of solid tumors associated with Hodgkin's disease [a]

Histological type / Location of secondary cancer	Epithelioma	Adenocarcinoma
Breast	1	1
Lung	1	1
Thyroid	—	2
Rectum	—	1
Tonsil	1	—
Pancreas	—	1
Larynx	1	—
Testis	1	—
Total	5	6

[a] Experience of Hôpital St. Louis (J. BERNARD).

Table 8. Therapeutic agents involved in occurrence of second neoplasia in Hodgkin's disease [a]

Therapeutic intensity / Second neoplasia	Mild	Intensive			Total
	Chemo- and/or radiotherapy	Radio-therapy	Chemo-therapy	Radiotherapy and chemotherapy	
Acute leukemia	1		3	2	6
Kaposi's sarcoma				2	2
Epithelioma	1		3		4
Adenocarcinoma	1	1	3	1	6
Total	3	1	9	5	18

[a] Experience of Hôpital St. Louis (J. BERNARD).

5. Possible Carcinogenic Drugs Among Chemotherapeutic Agents

As shown in Table 10, 3 out of the 5 patients who only received chemotherapy were treated with one drug — thio-tepa. One developed leukemia, the two others a visceral cancer. It is interesting to note that of the two remaining chemotherapy cases, treatment consisted only of MOPP, and that these patients developed secondarily a visceral cancer. Of the 18 patients treated with radiotherapy and chemotherapy, 12 received alkylating agents (cyclophosphamide, chlorambucil, thio-tepa, or TEM). For the other 6 patients the treatment consisted of a combination of drugs (MOPP, prednisone, procarbazine, and/or vinblastine).

Discussion

Even though the carcinogenic effect of radiation has been well demonstrated in animals and man, it is more difficult to incriminate with certainty that one anti-cancer chemotherapeutic agent is carcinogenic. In spite of the great number of pub-

Table 9. Delay of second neoplasia occurrence according to therapeutic agent and diagnosis in 24 patients with Hodgkin's disease [a]

Treatment	Mild Chemo- and/ or radiotherapy	Intensive radiotherapy	Intensive chemotherapy	Intensive Chemo- and radiotherapy
Delay (median) (years)		8.5	6.5	3.75 [b]
6	0.2—31	5—12	1—12	0.5—7

Diagnosis	AML	Kaposi's sarcoma	Epithelioma	Adenocarcinoma
Delay (mean) (years)	6.8		5.2	5
6	0.5—12	5 and 19	1—9	2—12

[a] Combined experience of Hôpital St. Louis (J. BERNARD) and Villejuif (G. MATHÉ).
[b] Significantly different from intensive radiotherapy; $p < 0.05$.

Table 10. Possible therapeutic agents involved in the occurrence of a second neoplasm [a]

	Radiotherapy alone	Chemotherapy alone	Radiotherapy and chemotherapy		Total
			Known drugs involved in human cancerogenesis [b]	Other drugs [c]	
AML	4	1 [d]	5	3	13
Solid tumors	1	4 [e]	7	3	15
Total	5	5	12	6	28

[a] Combined experience of Hôpital St. Louis (J. BERNARD) and Villejuif (G. MATHÉ).
[b] Cyclophosphamide; Chlorambucil; Thio-tepa; TEM (alone or in combination with other drugs).
[c] MOPP alone or Prednisone, HN_2, VLB ...
[d] Thio-tepa alone.
[e] Thio-tepa (2), Prednisone, HN_2, VLB (2).

lished reports concerning this problem, very often the absence of reliable statistics prevents one from concluding the relationship between the cause and the effect of the therapeutic agent (BELPOMME *et al.*, 1972). In addition, frequently many different anticancer agents are used, simultaneously or in sequential combination.

In our study, radiotherapy or chemotherapy alone was delivered in only 10 patients out of 28 patients. Incidentally, in 3 cases thio-tepa was given as the sole drug

(Table 10). Another difficult situation arises from the relatively long latent period preceding the clinical detection of the second cancer. In our study, a shorter delay seemed to be related to a combination of chemotherapy and radiotherapy and the occurrence of the second cancer seems to depend on the intensity of the treatment. This preliminary result requires confirmation, since the exact mechanism of leucemogenesis and carcinogenesis secondary to these treatments is still not clear (Arseneau *et al.*, 1972; Crosby, 1969; Jacquillat *et al.*, 1973; Powers and Poineroy, 1958). Finally, other factors such as a deficiency of the immunosurveillance could be involved in our patients and explain the occurrence of the second cancer or leukemia (Gatti, 1971).

Among the different types of chemotherapeutic agents used in our patients, the alkylating agents are the most frequent. This could be explained by the selection of the patients and the primary malignancy; however, the occurrence of second cancer in 3 patients treated only with thio-tepa is suggestive of possible carcinogenic effect.

In other studies (Arseneau *et al.*, 1972) as well as ours, the combination of prednisone, procarbazine and vinblastine may be cancerogenic in humans. This remains to be confirmed. It is interesting to mention that procarbazine has recently been demonstrated to be leukemogenic in monkeys (O'Gara *et al.*, 1971).

Finally, it is of importance to point out that even though this study suggests that anticancer therapy may lead to the development of a second cancer, the use of anticancer therapy will continue to be necessary for treatment of patients with malignancy. The risk of cancerogenic effect of these drugs appears to be far less than the therapeutic benefit. In the future, however, attention should be directed towards the possible cancerogenic effects of such agents.

References

Allans, W. S.: Acute myeloid leukaemia after treatment with cytostatic agents. Lancet **1970 II,** 775.

Anderson, L. P., Anderson, H. E.: Development of basal cell epithelioma as a consequence of radiodermatitis. Arch. Derm. **63,** 586 (1951).

Arseneau, J. C., Sponzo, R. W., Levin, D. L., Schipper, L. E., Bonner, H., Young, R. C., Canellos, G. P., Johnson, R. E.: Non lymphomatous malignant tumors complicating Hodgkin's disease. New Engl. J. Med. **287,** 1119 (1972).

Auerbach, O., Friedman, M., Weiss, L., Amory, H. I.: Extraskeletal osteogenic sarcoma arising in irradiated tissue. Cancer (Philad.) **4,** 1095 (1951).

Belpomme, D., Blondel, P., Mathé, G.: Les cancers d'origine therapeutique. Vie méd. Canada franç. **1,** 140 (1972).

Berg, J. W.: The incidence of multiple primary cancers. I. Development of further cancers in patients with lymphomas, leukemias and myeloma. J. nat. Cancer Inst. **38,** 741 (1967).

Cahan, W. G., Wooddard, H. Q., Higuibotham, N. L.: Sarcoma arising in irradiated bone: report of 11 cases. Cancer (Philad.) **1,** 3 (1948).

Catovsky, D., Galton, D. A. G.: Myelomonocytic leukaemia supervening on chronic lymphocytic leukaemia. Lancet **1971 I,** 478.

Court Brown, W. M., Doll, R.: Spec. Rep. Ser. Med. Res. Coun. n° 295, London: HMSO, 1957.

Crosby, W. H.: Acute granulocytic leukemia, a complication of therapy in Hodgkin's disease. Clin. Res. **17,** 463 (1969).

Feingold, M. L., Koss, L. G.: Effects of long-term administration of busulfan. Arch. intern. Med. **124,** 66 (1969).

GARFIELD, D. H.: Acute erythromegakaryocytic leukaemia after treatment with cytostatic agents. Lancet **1970 II**, 1037.

GATTI, R. A., GOOD, R. A.: Occurrence of malignancy in immunodeficiency disease. A literature review. Cancer (Philad.) **28**, 89 (1971).

GHALIB, S. H., WARNER, F. D., DEGOURIN, E. L.: Laryngeal chondrosarcoma after thyroid irradiation. J. Amer. Med. Ass. **210**, 1762 (1969).

HEMPELMANN, L. H.: Risk of thyroid neoplasm after irradiation in childhood. Science **160**, 159 (1968).

JALOTA, R., EICHWALD, E.: Chronic immunosuppression and occult lymphoma. Transplantation **14**, 397 (1972).

JACQUILLAT, C., BELPOMME, D., WEIL, M., AUCLERC, G., WEISGERBER, C., TANZER, T., BOIRON, M., BERNARD, J.: Leucemies aigues, sarcomes de Kaposi, epitheliomas compliquant l'evolution de la maladie de Hodgkin: à propos de 18 observations. Presse méd., 1973, in press.

MCKHANN, C. F.: Primary malignancy in patients undergoing immunosuppression for renal transplantation. Transplantation **8**, 209 (1969).

O'GARA, R., ADAMSON, R. H., KELLY, M. G., DALGARD, D. W.: Neoplasms of the hematopoietic system in non-human primates: Report of one spontaneous tumor and two leukemias induced by procarbazine. J. nat. Cancer Inst. **46**, 1121 (1971).

OLDHAM, R. K., POLMAR, S. H.: Extramedullary plasmacytomas following successful radiotherapy of Hodgkin's disease: clinical and immunological aspects. Amer. J. Med. **54**, 761 (1973).

POWERS, E. L., POINEROY, J. H.: Comparisons of the biological effects of ionizing radiation and certain alkylating agents in cell system. Ann. N.Y. Acad. Sci. **68**, 702 (1958).

SIMMONS, R. L., NAJARIAN, J. S.: Immunosuppression and malignant neoplasma. New Engl. J. Med. **283**, 934 (1970).

SMIT, C. G., MEYLER, L.: Myeloid leukaemia after treatment with cytostatic agents. Lancet **1970 II**, 671.

STARZL, T. E., PENN, I., HAMGRIMSON, C. G.: Immunosuppression and malignant neoplasm. New Engl. J. Med. **283**, 934 (1970).

SWAAY, H. VAN: Aplastic anemia and myeloid leukemia after irradiation of the vertebral column. Lancet **1965 II**, 225.

TOTTEN, R. S., ANTYPAS, P. G., DUPERTUIS, S. M., GAISFORD, J. C., WHITE, W. L.: Preexisting roentgenray dermatitis in patients with skin cancer. Cancer (Philad.) **10**, 1024 (1957).

Prevention of Chemotherapy Complications: Time, Toxicity, Pharmacokinetic, Pharmacodynamic and Logistic Factors

G. MATHÉ

Institut de Cancérologie et d'Immunogénétique, Hôpital Paul-Brousse, Villejuif

> But one must be able to evaluate if the patient will be strong enough with the "regimen" and anticipate whether the disease or the patient will succumb to the "regimen" first.
>
> HIPPOCRATES

It is more important that the chemotherapist should be able to prevent the complications of chemotherapy rather than to cure them. Each treatment used routinely whether by a cancerologist or a general practitioner should have previously been submitted to reliable therapeutic trials. This reliability should not only apply to the average patient, but also to the individual patient who might have cirrhosis of the liver or be taking barbiturates, both of which can influence the antitumour effects and the toxicity. Any new drug, if it is to be used in clinical trials by the cancerologist, ought to have been previously subjected to preclinical testing on animals using all the modern methods (see MATHÉ and KENIS, 1973, 1974).

This article is concerned with scientific methods and the ethics and logistics of clinical trials in which the doctor has to remain with the ethical code of medicine, and yet at the same time have the objectivity of the scientist. This has been the subject of recent reviews (MATHÉ, 1973; MATHÉ and KENIS, 1973).

I shall only discuss here the scientific principles which can enhance the safety of chemotherapy, particularly when combinations of several drugs are to be used.

1. The Combinations

Chemotherapists have been inundated by a flood of papers advocating combinations of several drugs. I shall ignore those which give a single cyclostyled prescription for all forms of cancer, containing half a dozen cytostatic agents, 1 mg Vit. B_{12} and 1 mg Vit. C, the latter inspired no doubt by that best selling Nobel Prizewinner, Professor L. PAULING (1971). Unfortunately, such treatment has its tragic side and has been the cause of several patients being referred to intensive care units, such as ours, in irreversible bone marrow aplasia. I will only discuss certain drug combinations which at first may hardly appear more logical than those quoted above, have, nevertheless, obtained a good worldwide reputation, perhaps because they have been well publicized or perhaps because the results have proved fairly remarkable (although it has never been demonstrated by a scientific (randomized) trial that they are no more or less toxic than other regimes). These treatments have been based essentially on the additions of drugs with different toxic manifestations. Table 1 gives a summary of these toxicities and provides a guide to the "rational" with respect to this parameter.

But, before recommending a combination and giving it an extensive publicity, one should be certain there is sufficient reliable evidence that the treatment can be generally used in hospital medical services and in private practice. Likewise, one should make sure the results are true and have not been manipulated.

We have compared MOPP (methyl hydrazine, oncovin, procarbazine, prednisone (DE VITA *et al.*, 1970) to an intermittent combination chemotherapy based on the concept of recruitment by synchronisation (POUILLART *et al.*, 1972). This treatment consists of cycles in which vincristine is given for the first two days to cause a transitory block in mitosis of cells which were distributed in the other phases of the cycle. This is followed by procarbazine as a cell killing agent given for four days. This oncostatic is among the chemotherapeutic agents the most frequently active in Hodgkin's disease (MATHÉ *et al.*, 1963). Finally, prednisone is given for 2 days, as it acts on the G_2 phase. We have seen that the frequency of complete and incomplete remissions when using this routine was rather better than that obtained with MOPP, and also that the lethal toxicity was nil while that of MOPP is not negligible. As MOPP contains nitrogen mustard, a drug active on cells in G_0 (BRUCE, 1966; VAN PUTTEN and LELIEVELD, 1970; 1971) it is not surprising that this famous combination causes severe and sometimes irreversible marrow aplasia (Table 2).

The chemotherapist must beware of being rushed into using these combinations without taking due care. When it has been shown that a combination of 2 drugs is more efficacious on one parameter of a malignant disease, for example, the duration of remission, than each of these drugs alone, before being too enthusiastic for the new regime, one must be certain that the toxicity of the combination is not greatly increased. Such an added toxicity was seen with 6-mercaptopurine (6 MP) and methotrexate (MTX) which according to the Acute Leukemia Group B only slightly increases the percentage of patients maintained in remission compared to methotrexate (HOLLAND, 1971) Fig. 1): however, this treatment induces a considerable immunosuppression, as we have shown with a variety of tests (BREARD *et al.*, 1974) (Fig. 1). This immunosuppression is a probably explanation for the raised frequency of pulmonary syndromes most likely of infectious origin.

The combinations should be selected on a rational basis and the additive and potentialisation need to be demonstrated in animals, then by clinical trials in man, before being used in routine clinical practice. This especially applies to those agents which are not active when used alone on a particular tumour, but are added to the combination on the pretext that they potentiate or could potentiate another drug that is active when used alone.

Table 1. Different toxicities of the different drug

		ACD	ADM	ARC	ASP	BCNU	BLM	BSF	CAB	CCNU	CPM	DRB	DTIC
Bone marrow and blood	B. M. aplasia		●	●				●				●	
	Leucopenia										●		
	Thrombocytopenia	●				●				●			
	Granulocytopenia							●					
	Lymphocytopenia								●				
Digestive system	Nausea-vomiting	●	●	●		●				●		●	●
	Mucosal lesions		●				●						
	Diarrhea	●	●	●									
	Paralytic ileus												
Lungs	Fibrosis						●	●					
	Allergic reactions												
Skin and appendages	Hyperkeratosis						●						
	Necrosis						●						
	Hyperpigmentation						●	●					
	Allergic reactions												
	Folliculitis	●											
	Alopecia	●	●								●		
Nervous system	Paresthesis		●										
	Polyneuritis syndrome												
	Deafness												
	Somnolence				●								
	Psychic changes				●								
	Cerebellar ataxia												
	Orthostatic hypotens.												
	Liver				●								
	Pancreas				●					●			
	Kidney												
	Bladder										●		
	Heart		●									●	
	Hemorragic syndrome				●								
Other effects	Immunocompetent cells				●								
	Cushing's syndrome												
	Hypoglycemia				●								
	Hyponatremia												
	Fever						●						

Short term effects

E	EPT	HN_2	MCM	MGG	MPH	MTC	MTX	PCZ	PLA	TTP	VCR	VLB	5 FU	6 MP	PDN
		●			●	●	●		●	●	●	●			
	●				●			●				●		●	
			●												
		●				●	●	●	●	●			●		
				●			●			●					
				●			●			●			●		
											●				
							●								
							●								
	●														
	●					●					●				
											●				
											●				
									●						
								●							●
											●				
											●				
							●		●					●	
															●
									●						
						●									
															●
				●											
															●
	●														

Table 1 *(continued)*. 2. *Long term effects*

Toxic effects	Drugs			
Delayed aplasia	BSF			
Delayed thrombocytopenia	BSF	CCNU	BCNU	
Paraplegia after intrathecal treatment	ARC	MTX		
Amenorrhea azoospermia	BSF	PCZ	HN_2	CAB
Cataract	BSF			
Cushing's syndrome	PDN			
Masculinisation	Oestrogens			
Feminisation	Androgens			

(MATHÉ and KENIS, 1974).

Abbreviations in Table 1:

ACD Actinomycin D, ADM Adriamycine, ARC Arabinoside cytosine, ASP L-asparaginase, BCNU 1.3bis(2-chloro-ethyl)1-nitrosourea, BLM Bleomycin, BSF Busulfan, CAB Chlorambucil, CCNU 1(2-chloro-ethyl)3.cyclohexyl-1-nitrosourea, CPM Cyclophosphamide, DRB Daunorubicin, DTIC Imidazole carboxamide, EPE 4-demethyl-epipodophyllotoxin- -D-ethylidene (VP 16), EPT 4-demethyl-epipodophyllotoxin- -D-thenylidene) (VM 26), 5-FU 5-fluorouracil, HN_2 Mechlorethamine, MCM Mitoclomine, MGG Methylgag, MPH Melphalan, MTC Mitomycin C, MTX Methotrexate, 6-MP 6-Mercaptopurine, PCZ Procarbazine, PDN Prednisone, PLA Platinium, TTP Thiotepa, VCR Vincristine, VLB Vinblastine

Table 2. Compared toxicity and results of MOPP and sequential combination of VCR, PCZ and PDN (Hodgkin's disease, topographical form III and IV)

	Number of patients	Death by aplasia		Results		
		Number	%	% CRg [a]	% IRg [b]	% Failure
MOPP	27	3	11.5	15	23	62
Sequential combination: VCR+PCZ+PDN	33	0	0	18	42	40

[a] CRg, apparently complete regression. [b] IRg, incomplete regression.

The therapeutic index of recommended combinations needs to be known just as that of each of the drugs when used in the same way one at a time. If the toxicities are additive or potentiate one another, experimental studies, then clinical trials should determine whether the combination is of any practical value. In this way, the combination based on the blockade of cells in M by an antimitotic, followed by a cell killing drug acting on the G_1, S and/or G_2 phase, which is based on the idea of synchronization, but may work also by pharmacological potentialization as vincristine (VCR) applied before MTX increases its penetration into the cells (GOLDMAN and FYFE, 1973), carried a certain toxicity in the doses used in the initial trials (POUILLART *et al.*, 1972) but the benefits are so considerable, particularly to obtain

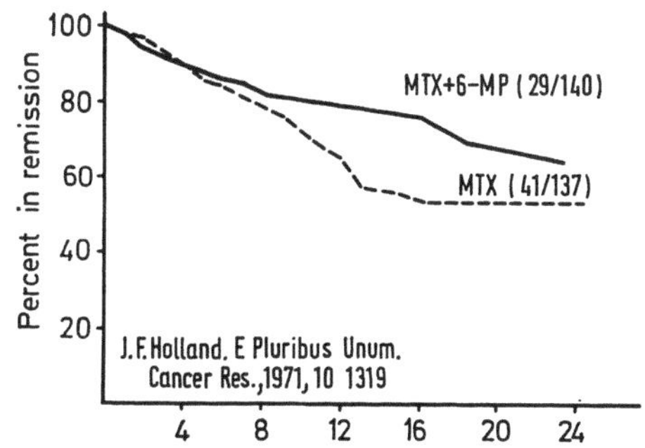

	in vivo [a]		*in vitro*	
	PPD Reactivity	Reactivity versus extracts of tumor derived lymphoblastoid lines	PHA Transformation [b]	Lymphocyte cytotoxity [a] versus lymphoblasts
6-MP+MTX	5/21	0/11	2/9	1/6
After chemotherapy	7/15	4/14	7/10	8/12

[a] N⁰ positive/N⁰ tested. [b] N⁰ normal/N⁰ total.

Fig. 1. The combination of MTX and 6 MP in acute lymphoïde leukemia increases slightly the percentage of the patients maintained in remission (HOLLAND, 1971) but is very strongly immunosuppressive (BREARD *et al.*, 1974)

remissions by the combination in leukemic patients resistant to each of the drugs administered individually (Fig. 2).

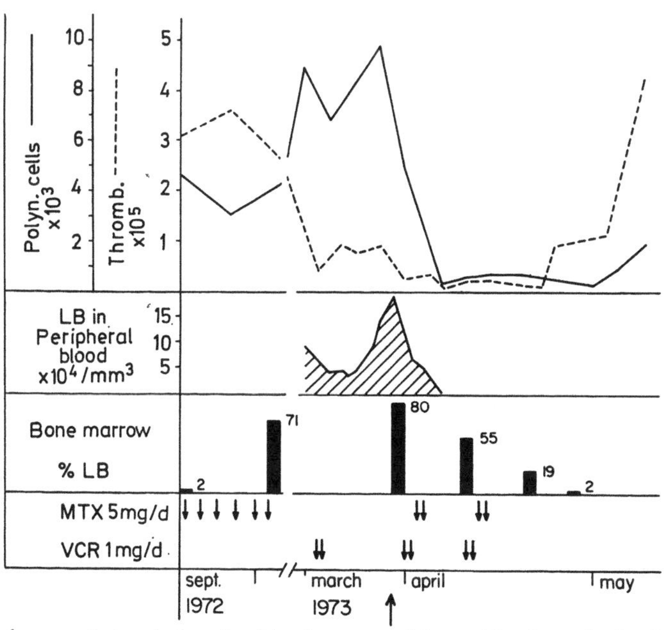

Fig. 2. Complete remission induced with the sequential combination of vincristine (VCR) and methotrexate (MTX) in an acute lymphoid leukemia patient resistant to VCR and MTX given separately

It is easy to reduce the toxicity by slightly decreasing the doses, or as it is an intermittent chemotherapy, prolong the intervals between cycles. But, in doing this, one allows more time for the tumour cells to multiply between the courses of treatment.

2. The Time Factor

In 1968, we observed (Mathé *et al.*, 1968), on L 1210 murine leukemia, that the same total dose of a cytostatic agent given once was generally more efficacious than when it was given in daily small fractions for 20 days.

This led us to propose the replacement of continuous low daily doses with intermittent high doses (Mathé *et al.*, 1970) (Fig. 3). The cycle or phase dependent drug or drugs should not be given again until the blood count is restored, that is to say when there is every reason to believe that the stem cells are no longer mobilized and no longer in cycle and have returned to the G_0 state.

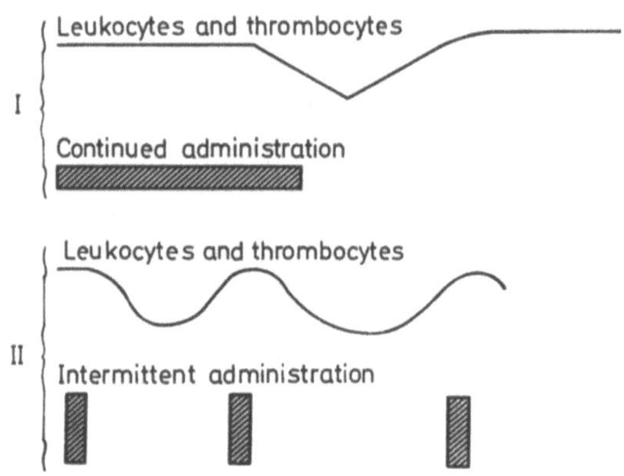

Fig. 3. Intermittent versus continuous chemotherapy

The fact that the interval can be almost of the same duration after each cycle is in favour of the exact hypothetical basis of this trial (Fig. 4).

A further basic argument in favour of the replacement of continuous chemotherapy by intermittent chemotherapy is their relative immunosuppressive effect. Most of the former are immunosuppressive, whilst the latter are rarely so, as shown in our own experience in Table 3 (Schneider, 1968; Mathé *et al.*, 1970).

There are two problems that need to be resolved for the further development of intermittent chemotherapy: how to afford the patient's complete safety during the first interval and how to shorten these intervals?

There are several answers to the first problem. Aseptic units such as the one we set up in 1965 (Mathé and Forestier, 1965) and have subsequently been developed in several countries in various forms (see "Aseptic environments", 1970) can reduce the mortality due to aplasia in the first cycle to nil, whilst it remains a hazard for patients nursed in conventional wards (Fig. 5).

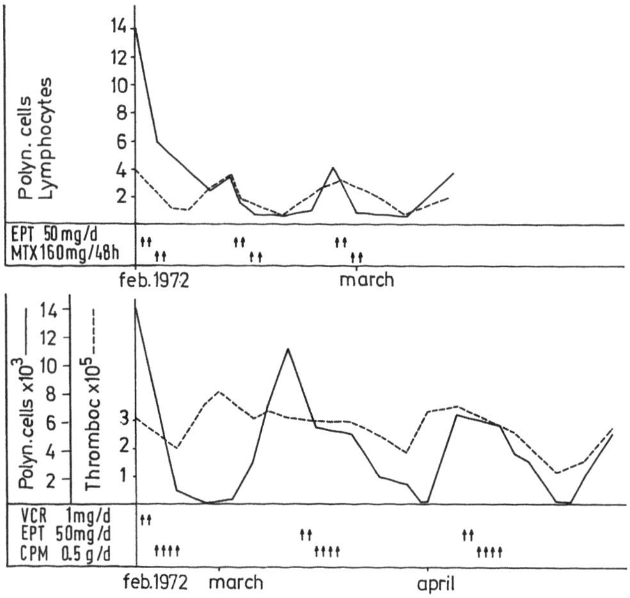

Fig. 4. Two examples of intermittent chemotherapy showing the constancy of the interval between the cycles

Table 3. Immunosuppression of chemotherapy according to the timing of administration

	Absence of visible immunosuppressive effect	Visible immunosuppressive effect
Discontinuous chemotherapy	51/57 (89.4 p. 100)	6/57 (10.6 p. 100)
Continuous chemotherapy	9/27 (33.3 p. 100)	18/27 (66.6 p. 100)

Leukocyte transfusions enable the severe infections complicating the aplasias to be overcome, in the same way as platelet transfusions can counteract hemorrhage complicating aplasia, particularly due to thrombocytopenia (SCHWARZENBERG *et al.*, 1966; 1968). Leukocyte transfusions have an even greater advantage as they can enable chemotherapy to be given to cytopenic patients and sometimes to obtain remissions (Table 4).

It is probable that under certain circumstances, the interval between cycles of therapy can be shortened. POUILLART and HOANG THI HUONG (1973) have shown that BCG and some other agents, in particular androgens, can induce stem cells in the G_0 state to enter the cell cycle. Applying this to attempts to shorten the duration of the time for haemopoietic restoration after a chemotherapy, we have seen that

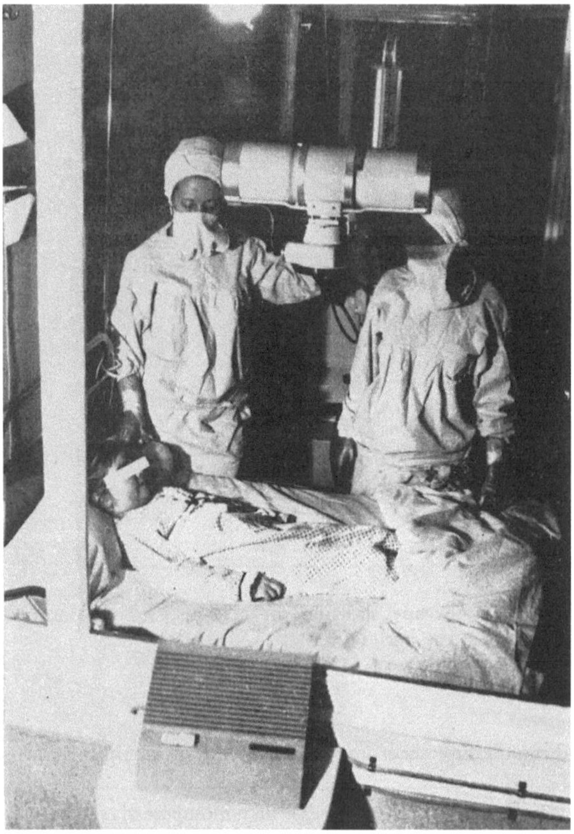

Lethal cost of first cycle:
Conventional ward:
10/200
Isolated unit:
0/50

Fig. 5. A room of the aseptic unit of the Institut de Cancérologie et d'Immunogénétique. The first cycle of intermittent chemotherapy caused no drug deaths in this unit, whilst they occurred when it was given to patients in a conventional ward

BCG, has this effect in mice treated with 250 mg/kg of cyclophosphamide (CPM) (Fig. 6 a) and in man given an intermittent chemotherapy regime (Fig. 6 b). In this way, by shortening the intervals, the courses of treatment are brought closer together and reduce the rise of the tumour cells between the courses.

3. The Antecedent Factor

A study of the reasons for hematological tolerance or intolerance during a clinical trial of VM 26 (EORTC, 1972; MATHÉ, 1973) has given some useful clues. In patients with initially cytologically normal looking bone marrow, we found that the hypoplasias were more frequent when they had previously received radiotherapy or chemotherapy and the aplasias (two of which were fatal) virtually only occurred in patients who had radiochemotherapy in the past (Table 5).

Table 4. Chemotherapy of acute leukemia made possible in patients with a neutrophil count < 800/cmm owing to preventive protection by white blood cell and platelet transfusions. No infectious complications in any patients

		Complete remission	Incomplete remission	Total failure
Acute lymphoid leukemia	Prednisone (100 mg/m2/day) Vincristine (1.5 mg/m2/day) Daunorubidomycine (20 mg/m2/twice a week)	6		2
	Cytosine arabinoside (50 mg/m2/3h × 8 every 4th day)	1		1
	Methotrexate (75 mg/m2/8h × 6) Folinic acid (25 mg/M2/6h × 16)	2		
Acute myeloid leukemia	Prednisone + Vincristine + Daunorubidomycine + Methyl-gag (200 mg/m2/every 2nd day)	1		
	Daunorubidomycine		1	
Acute monocytoid leukemia	Prednisone + Vincristine + Daunorubidomycine			1
	Cytosine arabinoside			1

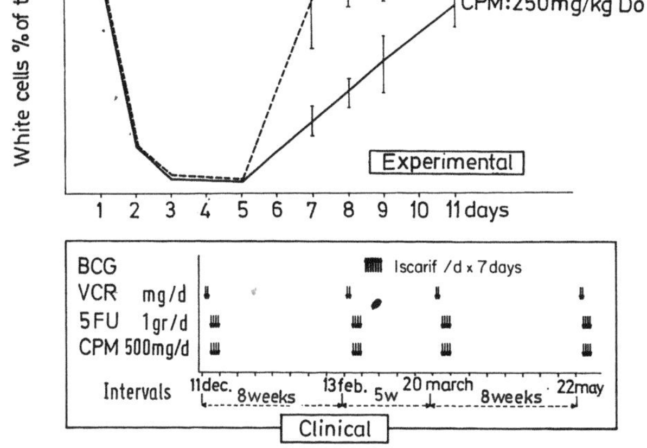

Fig. 6. BCG accelerates haematological restoration in mice after cyclophosphamide (CPM) administration and shortens the interval between cycles in an intermittent chemotherapy in man combining vincristine (VCR), 5-fluoro-uracile (5 FU) and cyclophosphamide (CPM)

Table 5. Influence of prior treatment hematologic tolerance to VM 26 in 60 new and previously treated patients with hematosarcomas

Prior treatment	Number of cases	No toxicity	Bone marrow	
			Hypoplasia	Aplasia
None	26	18	8	0
Chemotherapy	7	1	5	1
Radiotherapy	9	6	2	1
Chemotherapy and radiotherapy	18	2	8	8 [a]

[a] Irreversible.

4. Logistic Factors

It is important to pay some attention to the logistics of patient management. Thus a full account of past history of the patients' illnesses and treatments is required. Systematic questionnaires should be used in place of traditional history taking which the majority of physicians employ today. This approach is an intermediate step to lead the doctor away from old semantics towards scientific methodology.

The pharmacokinetics of the various drugs and their combinations needs to be the subject of extensive research, for it is only in this way their potentiations and antagonisms will be discovered. Pharmacosimulation should be available as, in certain genetic and pathological conditions, the effective drug concentration at a particular time can be increased or decreased ten fold, and thereby the effect will be modified.

To protect the patient against the short term risks, which are essentially related to bone marrow aplasia and immunosuppression, nursing in an aseptic unit may be required. Table 6 and Figs. 7 and 8 show the value of aseptic units. However, they should be more than just a room or an aseptic tent to show to the visitors. The unit's function is to support all patients who need aseptic environment.

To reach this objective we are now building, at Villejuif in the Hôpital Paul-Brousse de l'Assistance Publique, a Medical Service with a Microbiological Gradient.

Table 6. Efficiency of our isolated aseptic unit in preventing infectious complications. Incidence of all infections and of lethal infections in patients suffering from complete aplasia in acute leukemia

	Conventional ward		Isolated aseptic unit
All infections	94/117 (80%)		20/61 (33%)
		$\chi^2 = 75.0$	
Lethal infections	20/117 (17%)		4/61 (6.5%)
		$\chi^2 = 3.76$	

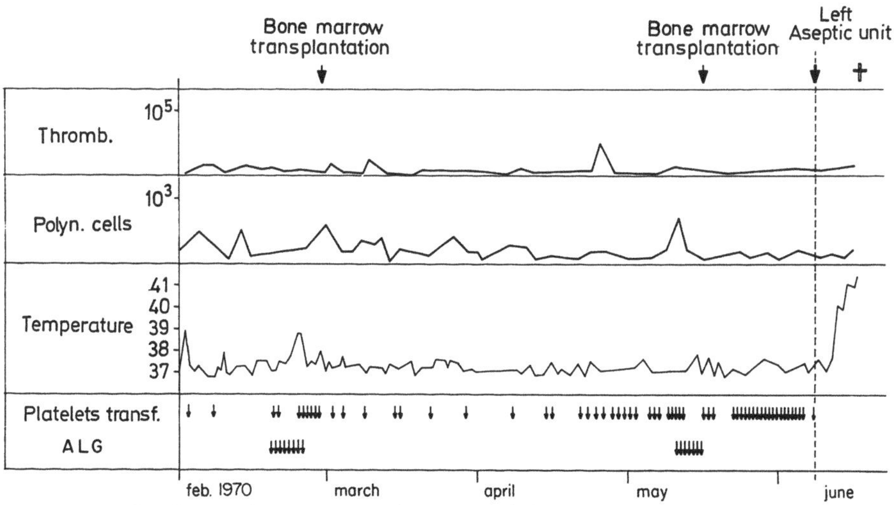

Fig. 7. Example of an aplastic patient who tolerated his pancytopenia while in the aseptic unit but who died soon after he left the unit

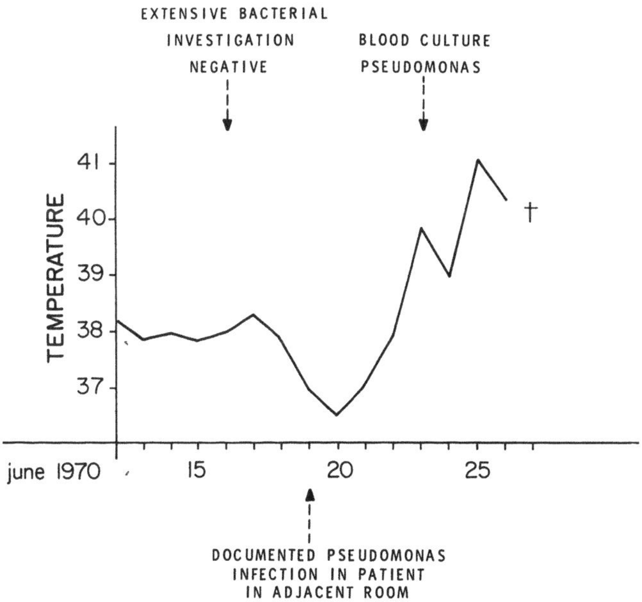

Fig. 8. Example of a patient who was tolerating his pancytopenia but died 6 days after a patient with pseudomonas infection was introduced by mistake into an adjacent room

This service will consist of a floor with a conventional hospital environment, a floor with a controlled microbiological flora and an aseptic floor. The microbiological conditions of the aseptic floor will be the same as those in the unit we have been running for the past 15 years (MATHÉ and FORESTIER, 1955).

Needless to say, white cell and platelet transfusions need to be available 24 hours a day and the oncological intensive care units should have access to banks of stored white cells and platelets. These transfusions are so effective nowadays that the indications for autologous or allogeneic bone marrow grafts (MATHÉ *et al.*, 1971) are disappearing.

In the logistic appraisal there are some factors, which unlike the preceding factors, have not been developed, but which have to be taken into consideration. The attitude of the doctors or the regional health authorities who do not always send their patients requiring intensive chemotherapy to specialised treatment services, but treat them themselves because they will not admit that they lack the necessary expertise. The requirement in some countries of the physicians to publish and their publications should give "good results". This can lead to a choice of a population of selected patients, choosing the optimum moment to stop the trial when the percentage of favourable results is still high, or a choice of a protocol which gives a high percentage of remissions at the price of a high percentage of lethal complications. It will be very helpful if the editors of scientific journals insist that the lethal toxic cost is given in the table of the overall effects of treatment, and a clear distinction is made between "complete" regression and "complete" remission (Table 7) (MATHÉ and WEINER, 1973).

In this way, the general practitioners who might be impressed by the high proportion of success reported in certain publications might possibly be deterred from prescribing a regimen which could be very dangerous for their patients.

It would be advantageous to agree upon diagnostic criteria, a nomenclature of diseases and descriptions of the results of therapy that could be used in an identical manner by different clinical groups and in different countries. A recent clinical trial on the chemotherapy of acute myeloid leukaemia carried out by The Leukaemia and Haematosarcoma Group of the EORTC (1973) indicates how this may work in practice. In this trial, the diagnosis and the "complete remission" were checked by a double blind method at the WHO Leukemia and Hematosarcoma Reference Centre. This led to accepting a much lower percentage of patients as being in complete remission than had been published previously.

There remains the serious factor of medical ethics of the clinical trial itself as it can be the source of complications that are often fatal. I have discussed this in a recent editorial (MATHÉ, 1973), emphasizing the role of compromise in the establishment of the protocol. This compromise can result in some groups of physicians giving doses higher than those which they could control the effects. Other groups would give doses below the effective level and they would be able to control the effects. This compromise can be satisfactory for normal patients, but is unsatisfactory for cirrhotic patients and those who take barbiturates.

Finally, the Swiss trial (BRUNNER *et al.*, 1971) in which patients with operable lung cancer were treated by surgery with or without complimentary cyclophosphamide. During this trial, the patients given chemotherapy relapsed significantly earlier than those operated alone. This trial went on for several years and raises the question of when to stop such a trial. To help with the decisions, many centres have formed ethical committees which, as present day doctors seem to be lacking in medical ethics, should have some non-medical observers.

Table 7. Necessary presentation for the first table of any paper on chemotherapy phase II trial. The lethal toxic cost should be mentioned in the articles and on the first slide at a lecture

Complete *regression*			Partial regression > 50%		Partial regression < 50%		Failure	Toxic cost	
With complete *remission*	With partial remission	Without remission	With partial remission	Without remission	With partial remission	Without remission		Lethal	Non lethal

To be detailed in a separate table

Definitions			
The tumour	Complete regression	=	The disappearance of tumour cells to the limits of clinical and laboratory investigation (Imperceptible disease)
	Partial regression	=	The measurable diminution of tumour cells by clinical and laboratory parameters (Perceptible disease)
The patient	Complete remission	=	The disappearance of signs and symptoms of disease to the limits of clinical and laboratory examination of the patient
	Partial remission	=	The measurable amelioration of signs and symptoms of disease by clinical and laboratory examination of the patient

References

Breard, J., Weiner, R., Oldham, R.: Immune restoration after chemotherapy and during active immunotherapy. This volume, p. 56.

Bruce, W. R.: The action of chemotherapeutic agents at the cellular level dans the effect of these agents on hematopoietic and leukaemic tissue. Canad. Cancer Conf. 7, 53 (1966).

Brunner, K. W., Marthaler, Th., Muller, W.: Unfavourable effects of long-term adjuvant chemotherapy with endoxan in radically operated bronchogenic carcinoma. Europ. J. Cancer 7, 285 (1971).

DeVita, V. T., Serpick, A. A., Carbone, P. P.: Combination chemotherapy in the treatment of advanced Hodgkin's disease. Ann. intern. Med. **73**, 881 (1970).

E.O.R.T.C. Clinical screening of epipodophyllotoxin VM 26 in malignant lymphomas and solid tumours. Brit. med. J. **1972 I**, 744.

E.O.R.T.C. Leukemia and Hematosarcoma Group. A comparative trial of remission induction (by cytosin arabinoside (CAR) or CAR and thioguanine, or CAR and daunorubicine) and maintenance therapy (by CAR or methylgag) in acute myeloid leukemia. Biomedicine, **18**, 192 (1973).

Goldman, I. D., Fyfe, M. J.: Free intracellular methotrexate (MTX) is required for maximum inhibition of DNA synthesis-augmentation by vincristine (VCR). Proc. Amer. Ass. Cancer Res. **14**, 50 (1973) (abstract 199).

Holland, J. F.: E pluribus unnum. Cancer Res. **31**, 1319 (1971).

Mathé, G.: Clinical examination of drugs, a scientific and ethical challenge. Biomedicine **18**, 169 (1973).

Mathé, G., Amiel, J. L., Schwarzenberg, L.: Bone marrow transplantation and leucocyte transfusions. 1 Vol. Springfield: C. C. Thomas, 1971.

Mathé, G., Berumen, L., Schweisguth, O., Brule, G., Schneider, M., Cattan, A., Amiel, J. L., Schwarzenberg, L.: Methyl-hydrazine in treatment of Hodgkin's disease and various forms of hematosarcoma or leukemia. Cancer 2, 1077 (1963).

Mathé, G., Forestier, P.: Un outil moderne de la recherche médicale française, l'Institut de Cancérologie et d'Immunogénétique. Intrications de la recherche expérimentale et clinique. Conditionnement hyposeptique des animaux et malades. Tech. Hosp. **20**, 47 (1965).

Mathé, G., Kenis, Y.: Logistics of therapeutic trials: the example of cancerology. Biomedicine **18**, 181 (1973).

Mathé, G., Kenis, Y.: La chimiothérapie des cancers (leucémies, hématosarcomes, tumeurs solides). 3rd ed., 1 Vol. Paris: Expansion Scientifique Française, 1974.

Mathé, G., Schneider, M., Schwarzenberg, L.: The time factor in cancer chemotherapy. Europ. J. Cancer **6**, 23 (1970).

Mathé, G., Schwarzenberg, L., Hayat, M., Schneider, M.: Chimiothérapie de la leucémie L 1210. Comparaison, pour sept composés, des effets de l'administration continue sur 20 jours et de l'administration d'une dose massive unique, précoce ou tardive. Rev. franç. Étud. clin. biol. **13**, 951 (1968).

Mathé, G., Schwarzenberg, L., Pouillart, P., Oldham, R., Weiner, R., Jasmin, C., Rosenfeld, C., Hayat, M., Schneider, M., Amiel, J. L., de Vassal, F., Steresco-Musset, M.: Two epipodophyllotoxin derivatives VM 26 and VP 16213 in the treatment of leukemias and hematosarcomas. Cancer 1973, in press.

Mathé, G., Weiner, R.: Criteria for short term results in the treatment of acute leukemia. In: Acute leukemias nomenclature, classification, clinical trials, methodology and actuarial results. 1 Vol. Eds.: G. Mathé, P. Pouillart, L. Schwarzenberg. Berlin-Heidelberg: Springer 1973.

Pauling, L.: Vitamin C and the common cold. 1 Vol., New York: Freeman 1971.

Pouillart, P., Hoang Thi Huong, T.: Putting mouse cells into cycle (CFUs) by diverse agents: radiations, cytostatics, androgens and BCG. Exp. Haemat. 1973 (in press).

Pouillart, P., Schwarzenberg, L., Mathé, G., Schneider, M., Jasmin, C., Hayat, M., Weiner, R., de Vassal, F., Amiel, J. L., Beyer, H. P., Fajbisowicz, S.: Essai clinique de combinaisons chimiothérapiques basées sur la notion de tentative de synchronisation

cellulaire. Administration première d'un antimitotique suivie de l'application de produit(s) cycle ou phase dépendant(s). Nouv. Press. méd. 1, 1757 (1972).
Recent Results in Cancer Research, Vol. 1. Aseptic environments and cancer treatment. Ed.. G. MATHÉ. Heidelberg: Springer 1970.
SCHNEIDER, M.: Effet des chimiothérapies antimitotiques sur une réaction d'hypersensibilité retardée. Rev. franç. Étud. clin. biol., 13, 877 (1968).
SCHWARZENBERG, L., CATTAN, A., SCHNEIDER, M., SCHLUMBERGER, J. R., AMIEL, J. L., MATHÉ, G.: Réanimation hématologique. I. Correction des troubles graves de la lignée érythrocytaire et des désordres de la coagulation. Presse méd. 74, 969 (1966).
SCHWARZENBERG, L., CATTAN, A., SCHNEIDER, M., SCHLUMBERGER, J. R., AMIEL, J. L., MATHÉ, G.: Réanimation hématologique. II. Correction des désordres graves des leucocytes et des immunoglobulines. La greffe de moelle osseuse. Presse méd. 74, 1061 (1966).
VAN PUTTEN, L. M., LELIEVELD, P.: Factors determining cell killing by chemotherapeutic agents in vivo. I. Cyclophosphamide. Europ. J. Cancer 6, 213 (1970).
VAN PUTTEN, L. M., LELIEVELD, P.: Factors determining cell killing by chemotherapeutic agents in vivo. II. Melphalan, chlorambucil and nitrogen mustard. Europ. J. Cancer 7, 11 (1971).

Recent Results in Cancer Research

Sponsored by the Swiss League against Cancer. Editor in chief: P. Rentchnick, Genève

1 Schindler, R.: Die tierische Zelle in Zellkultur. Geb. DM 19,80; US $ 8.10
2 Neuroblastomas — Biochemical Studies. Edited by C. Bohuon, (Symposium). Cloth DM 19,80; US $ 8.10
3 Hueper, W. C.: Occupational and Environmental Cancers of the Respiratory System. Cloth DM 41,00; US $ 16.80
4 Goldman, L.: Laser Cancer Research. Cloth DM 19,80; US $ 8.10
5 Metcalf, D.: The Thymus. Its Role in Immune Responses, Leukaemia Development and Carcinogenesis. Cloth DM 29,00; US $ 11.90
6 Malignant Transformation by Viruses. Edited by W. H. Kirsten, (Symposium). Cloth DM 39,00; US $ 16.00
7 Moertel, Ch. G.: Multiple Primary Malignant Neoplasms. Their Incidence and Significance. Cloth DM 22,00; US $ 9.00
8 New Trends in the Treatment of Cancer. Edited by L. Manuila, S. Moles, and P. Rentchnick. Cloth DM 39,00; US $ 16.00
9 Lindenmann, J., and P. A. Klein: Immunological Aspects of Viral Oncolysis. Cloth DM 22,00; US $ 9.00
10 Nelson, R. S.: Radioactive Phosphorus in the Diagnosis of Gastrointestinal Cancer. Cloth DM 19,00; US $ 7.80
11 Freeman, R. G., and J. M. Knox: Treatment of Skin Cancer. Cloth DM 19,00; US $ 7.80
12 Lynch, H. T.: Hereditary Factors in Carcinoma. Cloth DM 29,00; US $ 11.90
13 Tumours in Children. Edited by H. B. Marsden and J. K. Steward. Cloth DM 87,00; US $ 35.50
14 Odartchenko, N.: Production Cellulaire Erythropoiétique. Relié DM 34,00; US $ 13.90
15 Sokoloff, B.: Carcinoid and Serotonin. Cloth DM 29,00; US $ 11.90
16 Jacobs, M. L.: Malignant Lymphomas and Their Management. Cloth DM 22,00; US $ 9.00
17 Normal and Malignant Cell Growth. Edited by R. J. M. Fry, M. L. Griem, and W. H. Kirsten (Symposium). Cloth DM 63,00; US $ 25.70
18 Anglesio, E.: The Treatment of Hodgkin's Disease. Cloth DM 26,50; US $ 10.90
19 Bannasch, P.: The Cytoplasm of Hepatocytes during Carcinogenesis. Electron- and Lightmicroscopical Investigations of the Nitrosomorpholine-intoxicated Rat Liver. Cloth DM 35,50; US $ 14.50
20 Rubidomycin. A new Agent against Cancer. Edited by J. Bernard, R. Paul, M. Boiron, C. Jacquillat, and R. Maral. Cloth DM 53,00; US $ 21.70
21 Scientific Basis of Cancer Chemotherapy. Edited by G. Mathé (Symposium). Cloth DM 31,00; US $ 12.70
22 Koldovský, P.: Tumor Specific Transplantation Antigen. Cloth DM 26,50; US $ 10.90
23 Fuchs, W. A., J. W. Davidson, and H. W. Fischer: Lymphography in Cancer. With contributions by G. Jantet and H. Rösler. Cloth DM 84,00; US $ 34.30
24 Hayward, J. L.: Hormones and Human Breast Cancer. An Account of 15 Years Study. Cloth DM 37,50; US $ 15.30
25 Roy-Burman, P.: Analogues of Nucleic Acid Components. Mechanisms of Action. Cloth DM 31,00; US $ 12.70
26 Tumors of the Liver. Edited by G. T. Pack and A. H. Islami. Cloth DM 62,00; US $ 25.30
27 Szymendera, J.: Bone Mineral Metabolism in Cancer. Cloth DM 35,50; US $ 14.50
28 Meek, E. S.: Antitumour and Antiviral Substances of Natural Origin. Cloth DM 18,00; US $ 7.40
29 Aseptic Environments and Cancer Treatment. Edited by G. Mathé (Symposium). Cloth DM 24,50; US $ 10.00
30 Advances in the Treatment of Acute (Blastic) Leukemias. Edited by G. Mathé (Symposium). Cloth DM 42,00; US $ 17.20
31 Denoix, P.: Treatment of Malignant Breast Tumors. Indications and Results. Cloth DM 53,00; US $ 21.70

32 Nelson, R. S.: Endoscopy in Gastric Cancer. Cloth DM 53,00; US $ 21.70

33 Experimental and Clinical Effects of L-Asparaginase. Edited by E. Grundmann and H. F. Oettgen (Symposium). Cloth DM 64,00; US $ 26.20

34 Chemistry and Biological Actions of 4-Nitroquinoline 1-Oxide. Edited by H. Endo, T. Ono, and T. Sugimura. Cloth DM 36,—; US $ 14.70

35 Penn, I.: Malignant Tumors in Organ Transplant Recipients. Cloth DM 26,50; US $ 10.90

36 Current Concepts in the Management of Lymphoma and Leukemia. Edited by J. E. Ultmann, M. L. Griem, W. H. Kirsten, and R. W. Wissler (Symposium). Cloth DM 48,—; US $ 19.60

37 Chiappa, S., R. Musumeci, and C. Uslenghi: Endolymphatic Radiotherapy in Malignant Lymphomas. With contributions by G. Bonadonna, B. Damascelli, G. Fava, F. Pizzetti, U. Veronesi. Cloth DM 48,—; US $ 19.60

38 Koller, P. C.: The Role of Chromosomes in Cancer Biology. Cloth DM 48,—; US $ 19.60

39 Current Problems in the Epidemiology of Cancer and Lymphomas. Edited by E. Grundmann and H. Tulinius (Symposium). Cloth DM 58,—; US $ 23.70

40 Langley, F. A., A. C. Crompton: Epithelial Abnormalities of the Cervix Uteri. Cloth DM 58,—; US $ 23.70

41 Tumours in a Tropical Country. A Survey of Uganda (1964—1968). Edited by A. C. Templeton. Cloth DM 72,—; US $ 29.40

42 Breast Cancer: A Challenging Problem. Edited by M. L. Griem, E. V. Jensen, J. E. Ultmann, and R. W. Wissler (Symposium). Cloth DM 48,—; US $ 19.60

43 Nomenclature, Methodology and Results of Clinical Trials in Acute Leukemias. Edited by G. Mathé, P. Pouillart, and L. Schwarzenberg (Symposium). Cloth DM 58,—; US $ 23.70

44 Special Topics in Carcinogenesis. Edited by E. Grundmann (Symposium). Cloth DM 58,—; US $ 23.70

45 Koldovský, P.: Carcinoembryonic Antigens. Cloth DM 38,—; US $ 15.50

46 Diagnosis and Therapy of Malignant Lymphoma. Edited by K. Musshoff (Symposium). Cloth DM 62,—; US $ 25.30

47 Investigation and Stimulation of Immunity in Cancer Patients. Edited by G. Mathé and R. Weiner (Symposium). Cloth DM 96,—; US $ 39.20

49 Complications of Cancer Chemotherapy. Edited by G. Mathé and R. K. Oldham (Symposium). Cloth DM 58,—; US $ 23.70

Special Supplement: Biology of Amphibian Tumors. Edited by M. Mizell. Cloth DM 96,00; US $ 39.20

In Production

48 Platinum Compounds in Cancer Chemotherapy. Edited by T. A. Connors and J. J. Roberts (Symposium)

50 Cancer Registry. Edited by E. Grundmann and E. Pedersen (Symposium)

51 Cancer Chemotherapy. Edited by A. Clarysse, E. Kenis and G. Mathé.

Prices are Subject to change without notice

MIX
Papier aus verantwortungsvollen Quellen
Paper from responsible sources
FSC® C105338

If you have any concerns about our products,
you can contact us on
ProductSafety@springernature.com

In case Publisher is established outside the EU,
the EU authorized representative is:
Springer Nature Customer Service Center GmbH
Europaplatz 3, 69115 Heidelberg, Germany

Printed by Libri Plureos GmbH
in Hamburg, Germany